ABOUT THE AUTHORS

Zana Morris, a qualified nutritionist, is also one of London's most sought after personal trainers and has helped thousands of people get the body they want with her unique and effective method. Owner of three boutique gyms (The Library in Notting Hill and the Little Libraries in Barnes and Harley Street). She has over 20 years of experience in the fields of health and fitness and is renowned for her ability to achieve fast, effective results with her clients. She won the Best Quick Fix and Best for Rehabilitation awards in the Tatler Gym Awards 2014 and The Library was named London Fitness Facility of the Year in the London Lifestyle Awards 2014.

Helen Foster is one of the UK's most established health journalists, writing for titles including *Red, Grazia, Cosmopolitan*, the *Daily Mail* and *Stella* magazine. She has also worked for numerous international titles including *Viva* in Dubai and *Good Health*, *New Idea* and *WHO* in Australia. Her blog Health-e-Helen (healthehelen.wordpress.com) received the Highly Commended Award for Best Health Blog in the 2014 UK National Blog Awards. This is her eleventh book.

To find out more visit www.highfatdiet.co.uk

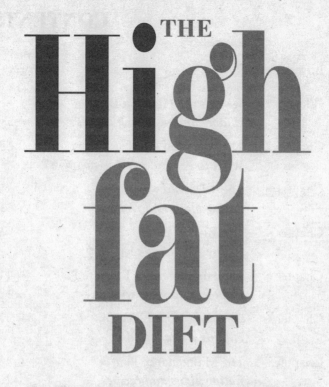

THE High g fat DIET

HOW TO LOSE 10 LB IN 14 DAYS

Zana Morris & Helen Foster

Vermilion
LONDON

CONTENTS

1 3 5 7 9 10 8 6 4 2

Vermilion, an imprint of Ebury Publishing,
20 Vauxhall Bridge Road,
London SW1V 2SA

Vermilion is part of the Penguin Random House group of companies
whose addresses can be found at global.penguinrandomhouse.com

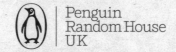

© Zana Morris and Helen Foster 2015

Photography by Nicola Bensley

Zana Morris and Helen Foster have asserted their right to be identified
as the authors of this Work in accordance with the Copyright, Designs
and Patents Act 1988

First published by Vermilion in 2015

www.eburypublishing.co.uk

A CIP catalogue record for this book is available from the British Library

ISBN 9781785040054

Printed and bound by CPI Group (UK) Ltd, Croydon CR0 4YY

Penguin Random House is committed to a sustainable future for our
business, our readers and our planet. This book is made from Forest
Stewardship Council® certified paper.

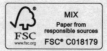

INTRODUCTION

Right now hundreds of thousands of people around the world have a common goal in mind: shape up and get fitter. It's a good goal – our society is in the midst of a crisis of obesity that's affecting our health. Shockingly, right now 65 per cent of the world's population live in countries where obesity kills more people than health problems associated with being underweight.[1] And yet, there is more information available about diets, nutritional supplements and medications than ever before, and going to the gym or taking exercise classes has never been easier. So why is obesity on the rise? Why aren't we achieving our weight-loss goals?

Well, it's not because of a lack of trying. According to research group Mintel, one in four people in the UK is almost permanently trying to lose weight.[2]

Let's look briefly at what we do when we want to shed these extra inches. Many of us start off throwing ourselves into it wholeheartedly – our diets change, exercise regimes begin and, if we're lucky, the pounds and inches disappear, but it is almost always a short-term success. Some of us lose weight then suffer the frustration of the pounds creeping slowly back on. Others, fed up with feeling miserable on plans that leave them hungry and deprived or disillusioned by lack of results, give up long before their end goal has been achieved.

The most successful dieters, however, find the plan that works for them. They stick with it, get results and reset their body in a way that means they keep the weight off for good. Sadly, however, these people are in the minority. According to one US trial only 12 per cent of people kept off most of the weight they lost for three years, while 40 per cent actually gained back more than they lost.[3]

So how do we lose the weight and keep it off? For many of you this book could provide the answer.

The High Fat Diet, developed by nutritionist and personal trainer Zana Morris, is a combination of high-fat nutrition and high-intensity training and for over 12 years has helped thousands of people lose an average of 6–8 lb (2.7–3.6 kg), with an average 1–3 inches (2.5–7.5 cm) loss from around their middle, in as little as two weeks. Some lose as much as 12 lb (5.4 kg). And, as the plan is designed to help reset the hormonal balance of the body, if they follow Zana's advice afterwards, it also becomes easy to keep it off.

But that's not what's surprising about this plan. What's surprising is how these results occur. It literally turns everything you thought you knew about weight loss on its head. Forget counting calories, feeling hungry, hours of exercise or months of watching the scales slowly shift downwards, and forget bran or anything else that tastes like cardboard. On this plan:

- You'll eat lots of high-fat foods – like nuts, seeds, avocado, butter and even cream cheese.
- You'll do no more than 12 minutes of exercise a day.
- None of that will be on a running machine or exercise bike.
- It only takes 14 days to get amazing results.

It sounds like it shouldn't work – but it does. Shortly we'll explain exactly how and why. But first, a few words on how the plan – and this book – came about.

ZANA'S STORY

I've always been fascinated by health – and the potential that we can release by optimising it. As a child, I loved health stores – they were Aladdin's caves of potions, all of which, in my mind, could cause magical transformations to occur. It was a seed sown by my mum who, in the days before the Internet, spent hours reading through volumes of health books. By the time I was 15, I'd joined her and was reading every book on health I could lay my hands on; by 19 I had qualified as a nutritionist and was supporting my studies by working part-time in a health store.

Throughout my late teens and early twenties I followed a great variety of nutritional programmes, exploring the effect they had not only on shape but also on mood, mental clarity and energy. Vegetarian, low fat, low protein, high protein, fruitarian (okay, this was only for a few weeks), water fasts... and finally high fat.

I also loved to exercise. Any exercise. Yoga was without question my first love, however I adored the intensity of martial arts, loved the challenge of weights, and with the occasional aerobics class thrown into the mix, I could spend up to three hours a day exercising. The gym was my second home – fine for when I was at university, but not always an easy balance once the real world of an eight-hour working day set in.

Then, one day, in my early twenties, I was asked, 'Do you train for health and energy or for fitness?'

At which point the penny dropped.

I was reasonably fit and lean, but had been blissfully unaware that the 'worked-out feeling' of which I was so, so proud, was actually a constant state of perpetual weariness, as my poor malnourished body was never given the opportunity to fully recover. I loved to eat – not recognising the discipline and willpower required to 'control' my eating patterns was stemming from a body crying out for nourishment.

It was at this point that I was inspired by a good friend to consider another approach. This was the 1990s and low-fat eating was at the height of its popularity. However, there was a small, albeit growing, movement worldwide that claimed fat was an essential nutrient, and that eliminating it from our diets was completely unnatural and went entirely against how we evolved. The theory made sense. Quite a few years earlier I had been introduced to the principles behind low-GI nutrition – avoiding foods high in sugars in order to keep insulin from spiking – and fat was an essential part of that. However, like all others of my generation, choosing to eat fat for healthy living and weight control went against everything I had been raised to believe. Nevertheless, I decided to try it.

The result was a complete revelation. Virtually overnight all my cravings and my need to eat copious amounts of food stopped. I no longer required willpower and a smaller plate to eat sensibly and well. I lost interest in snacking, in fact, if I did, I felt a noticeable dip in how well I felt. For the first time since childhood, I was no longer preoccupied by food.

At this time I was also introduced to the concept of high-intensity training. This is where you work very hard for a short period of time and allow maximum time for recovery and energy. That appealed to me. Even with a busy working and social calendar, I could still train daily, still have the challenge of an intensive workout, yet be in and out of the gym in less than half an hour.

I came to London in 2002, having qualified as a personal trainer. I started working from a small studio in St John's Wood, encouraging clients on to a system of low-carbohydrate, higher-fat plans for short periods of time, combining this with high-intensity exercise plans. I would get very strange looks from my fellow trainers when my clients left the gym less than half an hour after they started, but my absolute focus has always been results – I had little interest in simply charging for time.

Despite the consistency of those results – today we have over 400 clients per week across three different studios, losing not just weight but much more importantly, inches and fat – I have always been reluctant to encourage the general public into this way of eating. Apart from the public fear of fat, years of personal experience have taught me one thing: if you cheat, it can go wrong. Simply put, in my experience this isn't only the fastest way to lose weight, it has the potential to be the fastest way to gain it too! Fat is good, but fat mixed with any food you feel like is not. How could I encourage people to let go of the deeply ingrained belief that 'healthy' carbohydrates, from rye to fruit, are essential dailies, and ensure they stuck to this plan as carefully as they would when they were being monitored day-to-day? It was at this time, that Helen became a client.

HELEN'S STORY

I'm a health journalist and I first heard about Zana's diet from one of my peers who was raving about how easy it was, and how they could eat cream cheese, avocado, scrambled eggs with butter and still lose weight. I hadn't had full-fat cream cheese since about 1985!

I met Zana just before Christmas in 2012. I wasn't in the best shape of my life. Two years earlier I'd moved back to the UK from Australia and life had changed. I no longer lived walking distance from my gym or the supermarket so my daily activity went from one or two hours' walking a day to nothing, and the gym visits got less frequent too. I spent too many evenings exploring restaurants and pubs in my new town – and a lot of the time eating Cornish pasties on the train for dinner (you can't get a good pasty in Australia and I was making up for lost time). The result was that I was about 7 lb (3.2 kg) heavier than suited me.

Oddly, it wasn't the weight that was bothering me – I wasn't actually overweight, just not as happy in my clothes as I used to be – what was really making me miserable was the constant attempts at trying to shift it. Writing about health and nutrition meant I'd tested every diet going and, for me, cutting carbohydrates was normally a good way to lose weight, but this time it wasn't working. I'd start on a Monday, forgo all rice, pasta and bread, get on the scales on Friday and, when nothing had moved think 'Oh, what's the point?' then go out that night and have a pizza. It was exhausting, frustrating and miserable.

When I came back from a holiday and had gained another couple of pounds my weight officially tipped from 'I'm not happy' to 'I'm overweight according to the medical charts'. It was at this point that I knew I had to make a decision. I had to either decide that frankly, I didn't have enough drive to be thin and stop worrying about it, or I had to knuckle down and stick to something. The something was Zana's plan.

I was her experiment. No one else had been allowed to do the plan without supervision from day one. I had one session showing me how to perform the exercises, was given a list of gym machines to pick from and a diet plan to follow. Zana and her team checked up on me, but otherwise I was on my own. I admit it wasn't easy, I was extremely tired and felt rather sick, but the weight loss was frankly astonishing. A 1-kg (2.2-lb) loss overnight the first night and steady daily fall meant I lost 4.1 kg (9 lb) in 10 days. And 3.6 kg (8 lb) of that was fat. I also shed 5 cm (2 in) from my stomach alone – and, dropped 3 per cent body fat. Did I mention that this was in less than two weeks?

However, it was what happened next that truly astonished me. None of that went back on. Despite everything I had been told by Zana to the contrary, I was still expecting such a quick result to be equally as short-lived. I couldn't see that it could stay off – after all, none of the results of other 'speedy diets' I had trialled for articles had lasted that long.

A month later, however, it was still gone; two months later, still gone. And, other than limiting my carbohydrates to one or two meals a week, I was living a normal life. Over the next 18 months I had the odd gain when I went on holiday, but this time instead of those pounds staying on, cutting back for a bit would see them disappear. This remained the case until I went on a trip to the US and caused mass waistline destruction. This time it didn't go away again when I came back and started eating normally again. In fact, I started to gain again even when I wasn't doing anything to 'deserve' it. It was like I'd flipped whatever switch in my body had been keeping my weight down back on again – and it was well and truly in 'make Helen fatter' mode.

I cleared my diary for 10 days and went back on Zana's plan. This time I'd learned what worked for me. As much as I love oily fish like mackerel normally, combined with the high levels of other fats on the plan it was too much for me, so I stuck mostly with eggs and red meat. My fat came from a mix of avocado and cream cheese, or cream cheese and walnuts, rather than large portions of one source. Again, I lost 4.1 kg (9 lb) in 10 days – and again, it's stayed gone.

It was at this point I started nagging Zana to write a book. Obviously I'm a good persuader as – TA DAH, here we are. Good luck on your journey, I hope you're as thrilled with your results as I am with mine.

Chapter 1

WHAT IS THE HIGH FAT DIET?

Understanding why it works

Now you know how the plan came about it's time to explain exactly what it involves. We've told you that it's a high-fat eating plan, but it's also one that has a low-to-medium protein content and consists of very few carbohydrates. That means foods like cream cheese, avocado, nuts and seeds are in, as are red meat, oily fish and eggs, but pasta, breakfast cereals and fruit are out.

The diet plan is 14 days long in total – four days are a Pretox designed to prepare your body for eating more fat and fewer sugars than you're probably used to consuming and then the following 10 days are a high-fat blitz triggering maximum fat loss. Alongside that you'll do a daily short, but intense, exercise plan designed to not only help preserve the muscle mass dieters normally lose but also create a toned, sculpted shape. You'll also do some brain training so your mind helps you work toward your goals rather than sabotaging them. All of this combined creates the optimum environment for transforming your shape and keeping off what you lose.

Both men and women do the same plan, we just tweak it a little bit to allow for each gender. You'll get full instructions on pages 69 and 193.

HOW EATING FAT MAKES YOU THINNER

The idea of eating fat to lose weight probably goes against everything you think is true. For years we've been told that because fat contains more calories per gram than other foods (nine compared to the four calories in protein and carbohydrates) eating lots of it is the fastest way to get fat while cutting back on it is the easiest way to lose weight. However, as leading Danish cholesterol expert Dr Uffe Ravnskov said in his book *Fat and Cholesterol Are Good For You!* (GB Publishing, 2009) 'the idea that you become fat by eating fat is just as silly as to say you become green by eating green vegetables'. In fact there are a number of reasons why eating a diet high in fat can most definitely make you thinner.

Let's start with the most fundamental. Eat a diet high in fat and low in carbohydrates and your body has no choice but to start using your fat stores to fuel the tasks it needs to do each day.

The reason for this is fat's impact on a hormone called insulin. Released when you eat, insulin's job is to shuttle glucose, the sugar our body normally uses for energy, into the cells where it can be used as fuel. How much insulin you produce depends on exactly which food you consume. Sugar and carbohydrates (which your body converts quickly into glucose) produce the highest level of insulin; protein, which takes a bit more effort to turn into sugar, creates a smaller rise. Dietary fat, however, takes a few complicated steps to convert to glucose and therefore doesn't trigger any direct rise in insulin at all. Eat a bowl of, say, white rice and your blood sugar will rise quickly and lots of insulin will be produced; eat a pat of butter and nothing will happen to your blood sugar or insulin level.

Swap to a diet that consists of a lot of high-fat foods and very, very few carbohydrates and you create a situation where insulin is low and you remove your body's normal source of fuel. At this point it has to do something to get the energy it needs, and that something is to switch to burning fat instead (a state scientists call ketosis). To do so it reaches into your fat stores and starts to turn the fat within them into a fuel it can use for energy. Every time a little bit of fat leaves the cells to be used as energy the fat cells get smaller and lighter – and so do you.

ALL CALORIES ARE NOT EQUAL

Here's an interesting fact. When you start our high-fat 10-Day Blitz you could be eating between 1,500 and 2,500 calories a day (depending which meals you choose and how many of them) and still be losing weight, most of it fat, at an average rate of about half a pound a day (often far more), more than should be theoretically possible.

The reason for this seems to be something some experts call 'the metabolic advantage'. This describes the anomaly that when you eat a high percentage of calories from fat in a diet, you seem to increase the number of calories you can consume yet still lose weight. For example, look at what happened when researchers in the US put three groups of people on different diets.[4] One was a low-fat plan consisting of 1,500 calories a day for women, and 1,800 for men, two were high-fat, low-carbohydrate diets. One of these contained 1,500–1,800 calories a day (the same as the low-fat one) and one contained 1,800–2,100 calories (differing by gender as before).

What do you think happened? If all calories were equal, both the 1,500–1,800 calorie groups should have lost roughly the same average amount of weight, and the 1,800–2,100 calorie group should have lost less. But they didn't. In fact, both the higher-fat groups lost more weight than the low-fat one – six pounds more for the 1,500 calorie-a-day diet, and three pounds more for the 1,800 calorie-a-day one. Something happens when you eat lots of fat that seems to boost weight-loss results.

Exactly what that 'something' is, scientists are still attempting to pinpoint. Some say that because it takes more energy to create fuel from fat than sugar you burn up more calories when you start using fat as your primary fuel source. Others suggest it's down to eating more protein – you burn a high percentage of calories in protein trying to convert it to glucose, which reduces the calories you take in. While this might be true, Zana has found that on the 10-Day Blitz, the more you lower the protein content in each meal, the faster the plan works. She therefore believes it may be because fat also fuels fat-burning.

It's no coincidence that people call it 'burning fat'. When your body senses there's no sugar in your system it triggers the release of a hormone called glucagon, which in turn releases an enzyme called hormone-sensitive lipase. This prompts the fat cells to release substances called triglycerides – from which we create the final fuel we use for energy – and shuttle this off to our cells to be burned. That's right, burned – and what happens if you add fat to a fire? It flares, it burns fast and it burns bright. And that may also be what happens to your body when you eat a higher percentage of your daily calories from fat. It simply burns up its fuel at a faster rate.

THE FILL-UP FACTOR

Finally, fat also seems to make sticking to an eating plan just that little bit easier. Hunger is one of the main reasons people find diets so hard to stick to, but it's very hard to be hungry if you're eating just fat and protein. One reason is likely to be that ketones released as you start to burn fat for fuel suppress appetite, but there are many more reasons for the effect.

Because fat slows down how fast sugar is released in your system it doesn't trigger sudden peaks and troughs in blood sugar that leave you crying out for food all the time. Fat also digests slowly, meaning you are fuller for longer. It also seems to directly influence appetite hormones. Researchers at King's College London found that meals with a low-glycaemic index (which a high-fat, no-carbohydrate meal would be) increased levels of a fullness hormone called GLP-1 by 20 per cent more than a high-GI meal did.[5] Researchers at Purdue University in America also found that those eating a low-GI meal first thing in the morning don't just produce less insulin after that meal, they also produce less insulin after eating lunch too, balancing blood sugar well into the afternoon.[6] Can you imagine what difference that would make to eradicating your 3 p.m. energy slump and any subsequent sugary snacks you're eating to combat it?

Fat is also mentally satisfying. Humans find foods with fat some of the most enjoyable to eat and many people on low-fat diets miss the creamy sensation it offers. Called mouthfeel, this is one of the things that makers of low-fat foods try to emulate.

Combining the physical effects on blood sugar and the psychological benefits of being able to eat a food most of us enjoy can make diets containing fat more satisfying than low-fat regimes. This in turn can make them easier to stick to – and the diet that works best is the one you can bear to stay on long enough to get results. There might be one thing you're asking right now though: is it okay to eat all this fat long enough to get results?

Well, for starters, much of the fat you're eating on the plan comes from sources no expert is going to argue are bad for you. Avocados, walnuts, oily fish and olive oil all contain unsaturated fats that experts categorically state are good for your health. However, you are also adding in foods like butter, cream cheese, red meat and full-fat cheese, all of which contain the saturated fat those of us concerned about our health have been told to avoid. For a long time, foods high in saturated fat have come out as public enemy number one, but it might not be as clear cut as that.

FAT AND HEALTH – THE POTENTIAL BIG FAT MISTAKE

For the last 65 years, intake of saturated fat has been linked to a myriad of health problems. It's blamed for high cholesterol, atherosclerosis, heart disease, obesity and more – but what if it's not as bad as we've been led to believe? That's what a number of scientists, cardiologists and researchers are now suggesting.

This might seem confusing, after all, experts have been so adamant for years that saturated fat is bad, but what's emerged recently is that the study this view was primarily based upon may not have told the whole story. The study was carried out in the 1950s by an American scientist called Ancel Keys. Called the Seven Countries Study it looked at the dietary intake of people in seven countries – Italy, Greece, Yugoslavia, Finland, the Netherlands, Japan and the United States – and compared how much saturated fat was in their diet to the country's risk of heart disease. In Keys's eyes the finding was clear: the countries where people ate the most saturated fat also had the highest incidence of heart disease. Governments backed his findings and from this point on we were told that cutting down on fat was the key to protecting heart health.

In recent years, further analysis of Keys's work has found there might have been some flaws in the trial. Keys didn't take into account countries where data from other scientists showed an opposite effect to his theory – like France and Switzerland. It's also now known that not all of the data he used was collected effectively and that he didn't take into account other lifestyle elements – like exercise, pollution or smoking – that may have positively or negatively affected the heart-disease risk of the people he was studying. These findings created huge debate in the scientific community over what had been accepted as medical truth, so other experts started investigating and analysing and their findings have shed doubt on the idea that fat is as bad as we thought. In 2010, for example, scientists from the Children's Hospital Oakland Research Institute and Harvard School of Public Health examined the results of 21 studies that had followed almost 348,000 people over periods lasting between 5 to 23 years and decided the evidence didn't clearly support the idea that dietary saturated fat was associated with an increased risk of cardiovascular disease.[7] In 2014, researchers from the University of Cambridge analysed a group of 72 studies looking into the risk of saturated fat and heart disease.[8] Their analysis suggested the studies revealed no difference in heart-disease risk between those consuming the highest and lowest intakes of saturated fat, leading the researchers to suggest that we need to do more trials to confirm officially whether saturated fat is good or bad.

The sugar side of the story

Some other experts though aren't waiting for those trials. They believe the culprit behind our weight gain and poor health is sugar. Ironically, many of us consume more sugar since we started cutting out fat. Companies started to make up for the lack of fat in low-fat foods by adding sweetness, and we started to compensate from the hunger we felt by cutting fat out of the diet through snacking – most commonly on foods containing refined carbohydrates and sugars.

It's long been known that sugar was a risk factor for obesity and also that it was bad for our teeth, but now we know its impact goes further. Eating too much sugar raises insulin levels and increases the risk of a problem called insulin resistance, which stops your body listening to the signals from the insulin you do produce. This causes higher blood sugar levels, which increases the risk of diabetes. We also now know that sugar raises triglycerides (harmful fats in the blood that are linked to an increased risk of heart disease) and that it raises levels of the harmful LDL form of cholesterol. In April 2014, experts from the US's Centers for Disease Control and Prevention presented a paper suggesting that people who consumed 15 per cent of their daily calories from added sugar had an 18 per cent greater risk of dying from heart disease than those who consumed very little added sugar – and that this was independent of things like smoking or how much they exercised.[9] Such is the health concern regarding sugar now that The World Health Organization is proposing that no more than 5 per cent of our daily calories should come from added sugar in our foods.

Now, you might be wondering how telling you sugar is bad, or that a lot of scientists are a bit confused about fat, helps us convince you that it's okay to eat more fat while you try and lose weight. Well, it's because as the idea that saturated fat might not be as harmful as we expected gained greater traction, it became easier for scientists to study what happens if you ask people to eat more of it. Until this point it was either deemed not worthy of study or a little bit unethical. But since the debate began, the number of studies looking at what happens if you do eat a high-fat, low-carbohydrate diet, like the one we're suggesting you follow, has increased. What they're showing is not harm, but health benefits. Here are just three examples.

Yancy, WS, et al. *'A low-carbohydrate ketogenic diet versus a low-fat diet to treat obesity and hyperlipidemia: A randomized controlled trial'*[10]

In this trial, researchers at the Department of Veterans Affairs Medical Center and Duke University Medical Center in the US put 120 overweight people on one of two plans. The first was a low-carbohydrate, ketogenic diet containing less than 20 g (0.8 oz) of carbohydrate daily and an average of 68 per cent of calories from fat; the other was a low-fat diet consisting of less than 30 per cent of calories from fat. Not only did 76 per cent of those on the low-carbohydrate diet complete the whole of the 24-week trial compared to 57 per cent of those on the low-fat plan, the low-carb group lost more weight (12.9 per cent of their body weight compared to 6.7 per cent). They also lost a lower percentage of fat-free mass. Fat-free mass is also known as lean body mass and, as we will explain shortly, is the very tissue you don't want to lose.

In regards to health, the levels of triglycerides in the group on a low-carb diet went down and while changes in levels of harmful LDL-cholesterol were the same between both groups, in the low-carb group levels of HDL-cholesterol increased. HDL-cholesterol is often described as good cholesterol as it actually works to remove harmful LDL from your system.

Westman EC, et al. *'The effect of a low-carbohydrate, ketogenic diet versus a low-glycemic index diet on glycemic control in type 2 diabetes mellitus'* [11]

This study carried out at the US's Duke University Medical Center was on those with type 2 diabetes. One group were put on a low-glycaemic diet, which has long been known to help control blood-sugar levels, the other group went one step further and went on a very low-carbohydrate diet with an average of 59 per cent calories from fat. What the results showed was that both types of diet lowered insulin and improved the volunteer's ability to handle blood sugar, but the results were stronger on the high-fat diet. Over six months the high-fat group also lost 4 kg (8.8 lb) more in weight and their levels of good cholesterol also improved more favourably.

Volek, Jeff S and Sharman, Matthew J, *'Cardiovascular and hormonal aspects of very-low-carbohydrate ketogenic diets'* [12]

This paper wasn't just one trial but an analysis of a body of work by two of the scientists leading the field of research into high-fat, low-carbohydrate, ketogenic eating. In this paper they look at nine of the studies they have conducted since the 1990s investigating what happens to the body when you cut carbohydrates and increase fat and sum up their findings. The diets in their trials contained between 60–64 per cent of their calories from fat and between 7–10 per cent of their calories from carbohydrates. Among the results they found the following:

- While the diets don't tend to lower levels of harmful LDL-cholesterol that much, they do increase the amount of helpful HDL-cholesterol, improving the overall ratio of cholesterol (something shown to promote good heart health).
- The most consistent response to this type of diet is a reduction in triglycerides – particularly if you add a fish oil to the plan.
- Another consistent effect is a fall in the levels of insulin and fasting glucose. On top of this, insulin resistance improves. This is very important in lowering risk of type 2 diabetes.
- Finally, not only did all of the studies show the diets triggered weight loss, that weight loss was mostly fat, not lean body mass, and particularly it targeted fat around the middle, the type doctors now know is particularly harmful for our health.

That's just three examples of published works on this type of eating plan. There are many more, and time and time again, they show the same findings: that people lose more weight on high-fat than on low-fat plans, and that the majority of the weight lost is body fat. They reveal that while levels of LDL-cholesterol rarely go down on the plans (and yes, one or two studies have shown a small increase), the levels of helpful cholesterol increase, creating a healthier cholesterol profile overall. Insulin and triglycerides also fall. Right now, therefore, it seems that eating more fat and fewer carbohydrates while you try and lose weight not only works, it works without harming your heart health.

ONE WORD OF WARNING

While overall evidence indicates this type of dieting is safe, particularly in the short term, there are some people who shouldn't follow the plan – or should seek their doctor's advice before doing it.

Anyone with type 1 diabetes should not do the plan unless under medical supervision. Because eating a high-fat, very low-carbohydrate diet dramatically alters insulin levels, it's not suitable for anyone with this condition.

Those who already have heart disease, high cholesterol or high triglycerides should also not start the diet without seeking advice from their doctor. If they don't recommend it for you, this doesn't necessarily mean you've wasted money on this book. The Maintenance Plan in the second half of the book is lower in fat but can also help weight loss in many people. If they suggest you avoid the 10-Day Blitz, ask them if it would be okay to try the Maintenance Plan instead.

It's also not recommended that pregnant or breastfeeding women do the plan. Now is not the time to focus on any nutritionally restrictive plan but there's plenty of time if you want to use the plan later.

I've tried high-fat/high-protein diets before, why is this different?

Because it's not a high-protein diet. The daily recommended amount of protein for the average person who doesn't exercise is 56 g (2.2 oz) for a man and 46 g (1.8 oz) for a woman. This equates to approximately 280 g (11.2 oz) or 230 g (9.2 oz) of protein foods like meat or fish a day. For best results on this plan we recommend choosing the lower quantities of protein foods with each meal, and most people will drop to two meals a day – that means you'll be eating 270 g (10.8 oz) of protein foods at best.

Yes, for some that will be more protein than you're used to eating but compare with some popular high-protein diets, which can contain over 600 g (24 oz) of protein foods daily. These plans also usually contain lower levels of fat and moderate to little carbohydrate, which means they don't target insulin as effectively as this plan with a higher fat content. They also won't increase energy or reduce cravings as effectively and as such simply don't trigger such rapid results.

WHAT ABOUT YOUR KIDNEYS?

If you're eating more protein than you're used to you may be worried about the effect on your kidneys. Eating more protein increases the amount of waste your kidneys need to excrete and when high-protein eating first became popular some experts were concerned this might put the kidneys under pressure. Well don't worry – the largest, longest trial on this to date has now been carried out. Led by researchers at the Indiana University School of Medicine it followed healthy people on both a low-carbohydrate, high-protein plan and a low-fat plan for two years and found no noticeably harmful effects to kidney function, fluid or electrolyte balance from the low-carb plan.[13] They want to do a follow-up study on people with kidney problems or at risk of kidney stones though in order to check the risk in them. If you do have kidney problems, ask your doctor's advice before increasing protein levels.

Joints – and the risk of gout

Fats, in particular omega-3 oils found in foods like oily fish, are very helpful in terms of reducing inflammation that can affect joints. That said, there is concern that diets higher in protein or which put you into ketosis may increase the risk of gout. As you start burning fat for fuel, levels of a substance called uric acid temporarily rise – and it's the build-up of this that can trigger gout. On top of this many foods included in higher protein diets, such as red meat, shellfish or oily fish, contain purines, substances that break down into uric acid, potentially raising levels further – however, so do things you're going to be cutting out, such as alcohol! In all the years she has been offering the diet to clients, Zana has never seen anyone develop gout doing the 10-Day Blitz, however, she has seen many clients experience an improvement with joint issues. Leading high-fat, low-carb researcher Dr Stephen Phinney has researched the rise in uric acid that occurs during ketosis and he describes it as temporary and benign for most people. Exercise also speeds up how fast uric acid is processed through your system, so the risk of build-up is reduced on this plan as you are working out daily. However, if you are concerned, remember you can adapt any meal to use eggs or dairy instead of meat if necessary, but anyone who already suffers with gout should ask their doctor's advice before starting the plan.

GETTING THE BALANCE RIGHT

As we've said, on this plan you're going to be eating fat from a variety of sources containing both saturated and unsaturated fats, helping ensure you get a good mix of the two types. Many of these sources have health benefits of their own. Recent studies from Sweden,[14] Canada[15] and the UK,[16] for example, have recently suggested that saturated fats found in dairy foods may lower risk of type 2 diabetes; oily fish contain high levels of omega-3 fats that help promote good brain health, reduce inflammation and help your body respond better to a hormone called leptin, which tells your brain to suppress your appetite. Unprocessed red meat is a good source of iron that gives us energy. Add fat to meals and you increase the amount of antioxidants, like beta carotene and fat-soluble vitamins like vitamins A and E, that you absorb. On top of this, research has shown that vegetables consumed in the same meal as olive oil actually combine to create substances that lower blood pressure.

However, this doesn't mean that every type of fat is good for your health. Here are four that you definitely should avoid:

1 *Man-made trans fats*

These are types of solidified fats found in processed foods, particularly baked goods, snacks and margarines or spreads. They are one type of fat that we now know categorically harms the heart, as they actively raise levels of harmful LDL-cholesterol and reduce levels of the helpful HDL-cholesterol. The good news is, in the UK at least, most companies have taken trans fats out of these foods, but you do still find them in some imported goods. Read labels carefully and if you see the words 'partially hydrogenated vegetable oil' choose another product.

Notice we say, man-made trans fats. Natural trans fats do occur in small quantities in meats from animals that eat grass and in dairy products, however, their structure is slightly different and evidence has not found the same heart-harming issues with this form of trans fat – in fact, some studies have found the direct opposite, showing that intake of natural trans fats helped increase levels of good cholesterol.

2 Any kind of oxidised fat

If you've been focused on eating a low-fat diet until now you may not have eaten some of the foods in this plan for years. Maybe you have some butter in the fridge that you use for recipes now and then. Please throw it away.

Old fat is not healthy fat. When fat meets air a process called oxidation occurs creating harmful molecules called free radicals. Free radicals age our body and are potentially being linked to problems like heart disease and cancer. Reusing oils during cooking can also trigger oxidation. To avoid the risk of eating oxidised fats only cook with oils once and store them away from light in well-sealed bottles. If you start eating something and the fat tastes off, oxidation has most definitely occurred and you shouldn't eat it.

3 Vegetable oils

In the years where saturated fat has been the enemy we've been encouraged to consume unsaturated fats instead. These come in two types – monounsaturated fats like those found in foods such as olive oil and avocados, and polyunsaturated fats. Polyunsaturated fats can be divided further into two types – omega-3 oils, the absolute best source of which is oily fish, and omega-6 oils found in foods like nuts, seeds, margarines, spreads or vegetable oils. Both omega-3 and omega-6 are absolutely essential for health, but in excess these omega-6 fats can trigger inflammation in the body – and inflammation is linked to problems like obesity, cancer and heart disease. It's now estimated that the average Western diet contains 15–16 times more omega-6 oils than omega-3s when the correct ratio should be no more than 5:1.

One way to try and alter the ratio is to avoid eating foods like margarines that are very high in omega-6 fats and to never cook with vegetable oils like corn or sunflower oil. Get your omega-6 instead from foods that contain them in smaller doses and alongside omega-3 fats like walnuts or many seeds which help balance the ratio. It will also help to increase your intake of omega-3 fats from foods like oily fish and grass-fed meat.

4   *Non-organic sources of fat*

We live in a polluted world and we really aren't sure what those chemicals are doing to our bodies. What we do know is that these chemicals aren't all easy for our body to neutralise and excrete. When our bodies meet such a chemical they try and at least send them somewhere they can do minimal harm – and that somewhere is our fat stores. The same thing happens to animals. If you're eating high levels of animal fats, particularly if you're eating meat with the fat on, it's better to choose organic meats which are exposed to lower levels of chemicals during their life cycle and therefore potentially have lower levels of chemicals and other toxins in their system. We know it's a little more expensive, but if you can switch even just during the 14 days of this plan then do. Also, we do include bacon and chorizo on the plan. When choosing these foods try and buy brands that don't use nitrates – the substances in processed meats potentially linked to health problems.

On top of these last four pieces of advice, there's one rule you absolutely must not break on this plan and that is: do not eat any starchy carbohydrates, sugary snacks, fruits or milk.

Quite simply, if you do this, the plan will not work. As well as being the hormone that shuttles fuel into our energy cells, insulin also shuttles excess calories into our fat-storing ones. Start to raise insulin and, first of all, your body will stop burning fat for fuel and use whatever sugar it can find in your bloodstream, stalling your results – but if you raise insulin enough (maybe by sneaking in a slice of toast or two with your morning eggs) any extra calories you're consuming won't be burned, they'll be stored, and you'll start to gain weight.

Don't cheat. Don't cheat and, once again, don't cheat.

THE BENEFITS OF EATING LOW CARB/HIGH FAT

There are a lot of benefits to following the 10-Day Blitz

- You lose weight. On average people lose 6–8 lb (2.7–3.6 kg) in the 10 days – most of that body fat.

- You lose inches. Usually 1–3 inches (2.5–7.5 cm) off the tummy and waist and more elsewhere. This usually equates to dropping one, even two, clothing sizes. This is more important than any number on the scales – remember you're trying to keep muscle and lose fat and as such it's what the tape measure tells you that matters. As this is a very low insulin-producing plan you may particularly notice a real difference in levels of any abdominal fat that you carry. Stomachs flatten very well when insulin is kept low.

- Your skin looks amazing. Fat plumps up skin and by day 10 you could find your skin is glowing and fine lines and wrinkles have virtually disappeared. You'll also eliminate 'carb face', a light bloating that can occur if your diet is normally high in carbohydrates.

- You've broken your sugar habit. After the 14 days of the Maintenance Plan, when you taste something sweet it will taste very sugary – even milk in tea and coffee tastes sweet. By the time you finish the plan you could have switched off sugar for life.

- Your attitudes to food will have changed. You may have realised how often you eat because you're bored, tired or hungry. You'll also notice the difference in your appetite and cravings when you give your body a high-quality fuel of fats and proteins as opposed to the lower-grade fix of carbohydrates. Finally you will quieten that voice in the background that's constantly asking for the next snack.

THE EXERCISE PLAN

With all this talk about what to eat you've probably forgotten that the plan includes exercise too – but it does, and just as the nutrition part of the programme turns what you normally think about losing weight on its head, so does the exercise plan.

Why do we need to exercise?

While simply altering your diet can be enough to see you lose weight, it may not be an ideal solution. For starters, combining exercise and nutrition is more effective than dieting alone. Studies at the University of Illinois, for example, show that those who dieted by cutting calories 3–4 days a week lost an average of 3 kg (6.6 lb) in 12 weeks, whereas those who combined their diet plan with daily exercise lost 6 kg (13 lb) in the same amount of time.[17] Both sound good. But there can be a downside. Most diet plans don't result in pure fat loss, you also lose muscle. A lot of muscle. In the Yancy et al. trial we mentioned back on page 15, for example, the low-fat dieters lost half their weight in the form of lean body mass, while the high-fat dieters lost just 35 per cent. However, if you want to try and keep any weight you lose off, retaining as much lean body mass, or more specifically muscle, as you can is key.

Muscle gives you your shape, youthfulness and tone and, importantly, it burns calories – roughly three times as many per hour as fat does. From the age of 30, we naturally lose approximately half a pound of muscle a year – if you then choose a method of weight loss that reduces your stores even further things get even harder to maintain. The result is that many dieters regain all or some of their weight within a year or two and get trapped into a cycle of yo-yo dieting, losing weight then gaining it back, a pattern that becomes almost impossible to sustain. Exercise of the right type, however, can help minimise the amount of muscle you lose and hopefully even gain you some more; maximising the chances of you keeping off the weight you lose.

So what type is the right type? Well, it's probably very different from what you've used to slim in the past. Normally what most people do to lose weight is create the greatest gap possible between the calories they consume and those they burn. They cut back on food and increase the time they spend doing cardiovascular exercise like running or aerobics classes.

The problem with this approach is that if you do more than 45 minutes of training at any one time you can actually burn more muscle than you are capable of recovering. That's right: you lose muscle not gain it, reducing your metabolic boost even further. Our plan therefore doesn't use traditional forms of cardio – it uses strength training.

Strength training builds muscle. As you lift weights tiny tears occur in the muscle you're working. Over the next few days if you rest the muscle, these tears rebuild thicker and stronger so you can't damage them again – of course, the next time you workout you do exactly that, and as layer upon layer of damage and then repair occurs your muscles get bigger and stronger. Any standard weight-training programme will do this, however, what you're about to do is not a standard weight-training programme. We're using instead a form called High Intensity Resistance Training that will transform your shape in minimal time.

Quality not quantity – get results

First let's make something clear: you're not going to spend hours in the gym. In our plan you're going to be working out for just 10–12 minutes a day – in fact, the shorter your session (assuming your form is correct and you've completed it in full) the better your results. Sceptical? So are most of the people that try it, until they've done it.

High-intensity workouts, lasting 10–15 minutes have been validated by numerous studies as one of the most effective ways of not only decreasing body fat but also increasing muscle mass, strength, performance and endurance. This type of training can help to stimulate muscle fibres, increases metabolism for several hours afterwards and activates the highest possible release of a muscle-building and fat-burning hormone called human growth hormone (hGh).

When it comes to hormones and body sculpting hGh is vital. Produced by the pituitary gland, it's described as an anabolic hormone, which means it helps build muscle. It does this in both genders, but particularly in women. While men grow muscle via a mix of hormones including testosterone and hGh, research has found that women primarily fuel muscle growth via hGh. The higher your levels the more muscle you can produce and the faster your metabolism runs.

Because of its important role in tissue growth we produce our highest levels of hGh in our teens and twenties. At this point we make it when awake and asleep. As you leave your twenties levels start to decline: by the age of 30 some people won't be making any at all during the day and, according to research at Emory University Hospital in America, the amount produced during sleep differed fivefold between twentysomething subjects and those aged 60–79 – and not in favour of the older subjects![18] Exercise, particularly weight training and high-intensity workouts, trigger hGh release at any age. When it comes to producing the highest levels though, scientists say there are three key things you need to do.

1 Train using large muscle groups
2 Train at a high intensity – that means with heavy weights or at speed
3 Train with the shortest rest intervals between sets

So that's the type of plan you're going to be doing. No wonder you only need 12 minutes daily to get results – you're working hard and you're working effectively. But don't be fooled: just because it's short, doesn't mean it's easy.

DON'T BE AFRAID OF MUSCLE

Some of you might be getting a bit nervous from the talk of weights, strength and muscle building. You're probably thinking 'I want to be smaller not bigger'. Well stop that right now. The idea that you're going to look like Popeye if you pick up some weights is one of the most common misconceptions about resistance training. It's very, very hard, particularly for women, to grow overly large muscles – and it's impossible to do in 10–12 minutes a day over two weeks. It takes a very intensive weight-training regime and a seriously focused increase in protein intake, not to mention high levels of testosterone (that women simply don't have).

The muscle – or firm tissue, if you prefer – you develop on this plan, won't make you look bulky. What it will do is benefit your metabolism, helping you lose fat and it'll create a toned, sculpted figure that's stronger, healthier and fitter than one of the same weight with a greater fat percentage. Remember: when it comes to body shape strong has become the new skinny. Fit, healthy, athletic bodies that can do everything you want them to both now and for years to come are the shape we should all be hoping to achieve.

Because of this we won't be focusing so much on the weight you lose on this plan (although it will be incredibly motivating) but more importantly you should focus on the inches you lose and the dramatic changes to your body shape that occur. And on pages 30–33 we'll show you how to monitor these.

THE PERFECT COMBINATION

There's a term in science called synergy. Loosely translated, this refers to the fact that while two things might be good for you their power increases exponentially when combined. This is what happens when you combine the high-fat nutrition plan with the exercise programme you will be doing here. As we said, a high-fat, very low-carbohydrate plan aims to create a state where levels of insulin are as low as possible. An environment of low insulin is also what's needed for optimum release of hGh. Combine the two and you have the perfect combination for fat loss and muscle protection.

BEFORE YOU GET STARTED

It's impossible to know how well you've done at anything in life unless you know exactly where you started – and shaping up is no different. You're therefore going to want to take some measurements so you can track your progress, but you won't just want to rely on the scales. While you will lose weight on this plan, because you're hopefully retaining and possibly even gaining muscle, the scales alone won't tell the whole story. More important is the amount of inches you lose. So yes, record your starting weight but also get a tape measure and note down the following measurements. You will also find this form in Appendix 1 at the back of the book. At the end of the two weeks, compare everything to see how well you've done.

1) Stand on the scales and record your weight

Starting weight:_____

Finishing weight:_____

2) Measure around your waist at the narrowest point above your tummy button

Starting measurement:_____

Finishing measurement:_____

3) Measure around your tummy at the widest point, usually about 2–5 cm (1–2 in) below your tummy button

Starting measurement:_____

Finishing measurement:_____

4) Measure around the widest part of your hips – this can be lower than you might expect so move the tape measure until you are satisfied it is at the widest point

Starting measurement:_____

Finishing measurement:_____

5) Measure your thigh at the highest point of your leg just underneath your bottom. This is more easily done if you shift most of your weight on to the leg you are measuring causing the muscle of the leg to tense

Starting measurement:_____

Finishing measurement:_____

MEASURING BODY FAT

Surely if body fat is what you're aiming to lose on the plan, body fat is also something you should be monitoring? In an ideal world the answer is yes. The best way to measure body-fat loss is via what's called the pinch test. This uses small callipers to pinch different areas of your body, isolating the fat and spotting down to the millimetre how much you have lost. Done properly, it's a very accurate way to gauge results. If you have access to a personal trainer or someone at the gym who can do a calliper-based body-fat measurement before and after your plan then that's the absolute best way to track things.

Another measuring tool are the body-fat measuring scales that are sold in many high-street stores. While they aren't as accurate as a professional measurement they do at least give an indication that things are moving in the right direction – however, they can get a bit confused when you're eating a high-fat diet, so be warned.

The scales work by an approach called bioelectrical impedance. When you stand on them one sensor sends a painless electrical current up your leg, which then travels back down to the other sensor. The scales measure its journey. The more water – and muscle – you have in your system the faster and more smoothly the current moves; the more fat you have the more resistance it meets. Juggling those two figures allows the scales to calculate your body-fat percentage. However, the result can be affected by what you've eaten and they can mistake fat you've consumed as fat stored in your body. This can give a falsely high reading. If you want to use sensor scales, take your reading before you start the Pretox and then take a reading a day or two into Maintenance. This is likely to make it more accurate. You can record either measure here or in the back of the book.

Starting body fat: _____

Finishing body fat: _____

Ketosis strips

These aren't an essential part of measuring your results but they can be a fun way to check how you're doing and see how different foods affect you.

As we have explained, by eliminating carbohydrates from your diet and eating high levels of fat, your body will quickly enter ketosis – the state where it burns fat for fuel. When you do this you produce substances called ketones. These ketones can be measured in your urine via small strips of paper that you either dip into a sample you collect in a pot, or just dip quickly into the stream. The strip will change colour depending how many ketones are in your system. It starts off beige and the darker it goes the more ketones you're producing and the more fat you're likely to be burning. The idea is to stay in the darker ranges. If you tip back up to beige you've eaten something that will stall your results. You'll find ketosis measuring strips in pharmacies, or check Appendix 2, page 250.

Chapter 2

THE NUTRITION PLANS

What to eat and what to avoid

The nutrition plan takes 14 days and consists of a four-day Pretox that will begin the fat-burning process and prepare your body for the 10-Day high-fat, low-carbohydrate Blitz that follows. Here's an outline of both plans so you know what to expect.

THE PRETOX: DAYS 1–4

The point of this part of the plan is to simply get your body ready for the 10-Day Blitz. It might sound an odd thing to do, why can't you just get on with things? Well you can, however, years of experience have taught Zana that a sudden switch from a diet where your body is burning sugar as its primary fuel source to a high-fat, low-carbohydrate one, where fat becomes the fuel can, in some people, cause a few small side effects from sugar withdrawal or from your body being unaccustomed to the sudden increase in fat.

It's not surprising. Our typical diet is very carbohydrate and sugar heavy. Cereal with milk for breakfast, sandwiches for lunch and something with rice or pasta in the evening all break down into sugars in our body. On top of these naturally occurring sugars, each one of us normally eats around 12 per cent of our daily calories in the form of added sugars in foods like sweet treats or even savoury items like coleslaw, pasta sauce or ketchup.[19] Then there's alcohol, another sugar: 52 per cent of women and 64 per cent of men have at least one alcoholic drink a week and many of us have more than one.[20] Removing all these sugars suddenly from your diet can cause a form of withdrawal that can lead to fatigue and grumpiness. Not to mention, if you're used to sustaining your day with sugar you might find psychologically that not being able to reach for your fix can also cause a dip in your energy and mood.

We're also not used to eating quite as much fat as you'll be eating on this plan. The average consumption of oily fish, for example, in the UK is only 54 g (2.1 oz) each week[21] – far less than the minimum of one 140-g (5.6-oz) portion government recommendations suggest we consume. Many of us rarely eat nuts and even though 13 per cent of our daily calories on average come from saturated fat,[22] it's often wrapped up in the form of sugary treats that studies show actually reduce the taste of fat you detect. This can mean that eating the high levels of fat on this plan can take a bit of getting used to. If you're used to consuming a low-fat diet, the added fullness and the richness of the foods you're consuming, combined with the energy dips from sugar withdrawal, could make you feel a bit queasy. By going on the four-day Pretox you can avoid these possible side effects as you prepare your system for the changes in your normal routine.

What does the Pretox involve?

It's simple – you're going to stop eating the following foods completely to lower your blood-sugar levels:

- Starchy carbohydrates: that means bread, pastry, rice, pasta, potatoes, grains, oats, breakfast cereals, etc.
- Sugars: no table sugar, sweets, cakes, chocolate, alcohol or artificial sweeteners and diet drinks (see why on page 52)

- High-sugar fruits: like bananas, figs, grapes, mango, melon, papaya and pineapple, and dried fruit like dates, figs, raisins, sultanas

You're also going to gradually increase your intake of the following foods to get you more used to eating fat:

- Oily fish
- Avocados
- Nuts
- Occasional high-fat dairy like crème fraîche or cream cheese

But it's not just your body that you prepare during the Pretox. These four days are also the perfect time to prepare your cupboards, plan your workout and start some of the mind exercises in Chapter 6 so you know exactly what you're doing when the 10-Day Blitz starts.

THE 10-DAY BLITZ – DAYS 5–14

While some people will start to lose weight on the Pretox, it's this part of the plan that will trigger maximum fat and inch loss. For the 10 days on this part of the plan your meals contain only three food types – fats, proteins and vegetables – but as the success of the plan is based on how each of these impacts on the release of insulin you may be a bit surprised to see exactly how we classify these foods. It won't always reflect what you perhaps learned at school or what you have been told by other nutritional or health experts over the years.

Over the next few pages we're going to explain all of this. Don't skip this section. Chances are there will be some meals on the plan with ingredients you may not like. By using the information included in the next few pages you'll have the information you need to help switch things around throughout the 10-Day Blitz.

But more importantly, these pages clearly pinpoint some pitfalls that could stall your results during the Blitz. When it comes to affecting insulin, all foods, even from the same food type, are not equal. While, for example, a small plate of lettuce has hardly any impact on insulin, the same size plate of cooked carrots will raise levels considerably higher.

The most important section on the pages that follow is the foods to avoid. These are foods that contain some level of carbohydrates or sugar that can stall the plan and some of them may surprise you – Helen once called Zana feeling very confused when her weight loss stopped dead (after losing 0.5–1 kg or 1–2 lb daily in the days beforehand) only for Zana to ask her to check the label on the bacon she'd eaten last night – and yes, sure enough, it contained a bit too much sugar that had been added as flavouring. Zana herself got caught out in the early days by eating sugar-free gum. Even though most artificial sweeteners don't cause insulin spikes some, like xylitol, can cause a very small rise. And yes, a little splash of milk in your tea can matter. It's one of the most common things that Zana finds her clients have been doing if things slow down.

So, now let's give you the details you need as to exactly what to eat and what to avoid.

Fats

Unquestionably the most important nutrient in this plan, fat forms the basis of every meal and makes up the main source of calories you're going to consume during the 10-Day Blitz. In fact, if you're used to the modern low-fat diet you'll possibly be quite surprised by how much of it you are going to consume, but if your fat levels on the plan aren't high enough, your body won't get to the point where it uses maximum fat for fuel. Ideally, you're looking at a ratio of at least three times more fat calories than protein calories per day.

To be classed as a fat in this plan a food must contain over 70 per cent of its calories from fat and have extremely low carbohydrate levels. Cheese is unquestionably a high-fat food, but for the purpose of this plan we divide cheeses into full-fat cream cheeses and all other cheeses. The reason is that the ratio of fat to protein is too low in all other cheese. A serving of Edam, for example, contains 68 per cent of its calories from fat and 28 per cent from protein; Emmental gets 69 per cent of its calories from fat and 29 per cent from protein. Compare that to a portion of full-fat cream cheese which contains 86 per cent of its calories from fat and just 8 per cent from protein and you can clearly see the difference. On this plan, full-fat cream cheese and mascarpone class as fats, all other cheeses fall into the category of proteins, which we'll talk about on pages 38–42. The percentage of fat calories is also why we only allow certain types of nuts – the others do have high levels of fat, but may also contain a slightly higher proportion of carbohydrates than the walnuts, macadamia or pine nuts recommended on this part of the plan.

You'll note that we mostly talk about a whole or half an avocado on the plan, rather than having you measure them out. When we do this we are referring to Hass avocados, which are the small to medium ones about the size of your fist. If you prefer to buy the larger, Californian avocado, use half of one where we suggest a whole avocado and about a quarter when we say half. Don't worry about being too precise however, a little extra fat from avocado won't hurt.

Most diets will make the difference between saturated and unsaturated fats, perceived wisdom being that you should focus your diet on the unsaturated fats which are deemed healthier; we've discussed why this may no longer be the case on pages 13–14 but there is still a good mix of foods containing both types within our meal suggestions.

Pick those you are going to enjoy most but try and vary things so you get a good variety of foods and types of fat. All fats, saturated and unsaturated, have an equally negligible effect on insulin release.

ALLOWED

- Dairy foods: butter, clotted cream, crème fraîche, double cream, full-fat cream cheese like Philadelphia or Boursin, mascarpone, single cream, sour cream, whipping cream (no added sugar)
- Fruits, nuts and seeds: avocado, CO YO coconut-based yogurt (the natural, unsweetened version), macadamia nuts, pine nuts, pumpkin seeds, walnuts
- Oils and dressings: coconut oil, homemade mayonnaise, ghee, nut oils, olive oil

AVOID

- All nuts not mentioned above: almonds, Brazil nuts, cashews, pistachios, etc.
- Any seeds not mentioned above: like flax, sunflower, sesame
- Fresh coconut, low-fat cream cheese, margarine and low-fat spreads, nut butters, vegetable oils

Protein foods

After fat, protein-based foods will make up the next largest proportion of your meals.

Protein partners fat extremely well. It supplies nutrients that fat doesn't and boosts its satiating effects. In studies at the University of Washington in America, people consuming a diet in which their protein intake was increased to 30 per cent of their calories and 20 per cent from fat decreased their appetites so much that their daily calorie intake naturally dropped by between 380–506 calories.[23] One thing you'll notice on this plan is that you are never hungry between meals.

While all of these are great reasons to eat protein, its primary job on this plan is to ensure muscle recovery after training. Protein is the only food group to break down to amino acids, which are effectively the building blocks of your entire body. Essential to build all of your structural tissue from skin to hair, they also help you create firm tissue – or muscle – that you need to keep your metabolism high. Of all the amino acids what's emerging from studies is that one, leucine, is vital. Leucine seems to be the substance that switches on the process of muscle building. Healthy levels of this in your diet therefore help maximise muscle growth and prevent its loss while dieting. Leucine is found in foods like meat, poultry and fish, which you're going to be eating plenty of.

The types of protein you can consume on the plan fit into two groups – those that also have a naturally high-fat content of their own like sirloin steak or lamb, oily fish, eggs and cheese, which should be the types you eat most often – and lower-fat proteins which you can consume if you also add some fat when you cook or serve them. This helps ensure you keep that all important ratio of three times fat calories to protein calories.

One thing that you do have to avoid during the 10-Day Blitz are milks and yogurts as they contain high levels of milk sugars. We included Greek yogurt and let you have milk in tea and coffee in the Pretox specifically to help you avoid a dramatic sugar withdrawal – but for the next 10 days they are off the menu.

ALLOWED

- Beef: mince (10 per cent fat or above), ribs (no sauce), steak, particularly rib-eye or sirloin
- Cheese: any full-fat cheese like Brie, Camembert, Gorgonzola, Emmental, Gruyère, halloumi, Roquefort, Stilton or blue cheese
- Eggs: ideally organic. Hen, duck or quail
- Lamb: all cuts including breast, chops, leg, mince, neck, rack, rump, shanks, shoulder
- Oily fish: anchovies, eel, fresh salmon, fresh tuna, herring, kippers, mackerel, pilchards, sardines, smoked salmon, trout, tuna canned in oil, whitebait (not breaded)
- Pork: including bacon, particularly streaky bacon (ensure that there is no added sugar and ideally free from nitrates), chorizo (no added sugar and ideally free from nitrates), gammon, pancetta, Parma ham, pork belly, pork chops, pork fillet, ribs (no sauce), tenderloin
- Poultry: chicken drumsticks (skin on), chicken thighs, chicken wings, duck. All chicken should be organic

ALLOWED – WITH EXTRA FAT

Cook the following with butter or oil; eat poultry with the skin on; add cream/cream cheese

- Beef: less than 5 per cent fat mince, roasting joints, veal
- Dairy: casein protein powder, full-fat cottage cheese, reduced-fat versions of any cheese including cottage cheese

- Fish: all white fish like cod, haddock, sole, pollock. Tuna canned in brine or spring water
- Offal: liver, kidney, heart
- Pork: lean or reduced-fat mince
- Poultry and game: organic chicken breast, partridge, pigeon, rabbit, turkey, venison
- Shellfish: prawns, mussels, crab, crayfish

AVOID

- Beans and pulses
- Beefburgers (unless 100 per cent pure beef with no added wheat)
- Breaded fish products, canned fish products with any kind of sauce
- Milk and milk products like ice cream or any non-dairy alternative
- Processed fish products like crabsticks
- Processed sandwich-style meats, sausages, tinned meats
- Yogurt of any kind, including full-fat Greek yogurt

There are a lot of eggs on this plan. Is that okay?

Just as fat has been very misunderstood so too has the role of eggs and their link with cholesterol. Eggs contain natural cholesterol and it was once believed that this raised our blood cholesterol levels. We know now that that isn't true and they are fine to eat regularly. Eggs also contain many vitamins and minerals. One egg contains over half the vitamin B12 you need in a day, almost a third of the recommended amount of vitamin D and healthy levels of iodine, selenium, vitamin A and many other nutrients. However, we highly recommend you choose good-quality organic eggs.

PROTEIN SHAKES

These seem to be staple fuel for anyone who does weight training. They can be included within the meal options in this plan but you have to choose your brand very carefully. Many brands add sugars and sweeteners which will immediately exclude them.

The next thing to check is the type of protein the product is made from – there are a myriad of these available now derived from everything from whey to pumpkin; Zana, however, prefers casein-based powders.

Casein is the substance that gives cow's milk its protein content and it is the reason milk is white. It's also a complete protein, so very readily absorbed, and has the added bonus of supplying natural calcium. Most importantly, it digests very slowly and so has the lowest effect on insulin. Casein is fat free so, if you want to use it as part of the diet you won't be able to simply mix it into a drink with water or milk. Instead, try making it into one of Zana's mousses (see recipes on pages 89–90), which combine it with sources of fats.

CAN I DO THIS PLAN IF I DON'T EAT MEAT?

The answer to this depends very much on what else you do eat. If you are vegan, to be honest, it's virtually impossible to get the fat and protein ratios right and eat enough different foods to sustain you healthily for 10 days.

If you simply don't eat meat, but do eat fish, or if you shun meat, fish and poultry but eat cheese, eggs and dairy it's completely feasible. In fact, Zana has worked with numerous vegetarian clients whose diets had been based heavily on refined carbohydrates and very little protein and found they have transformed their bodies on the plan. All you need to do is use these pages to help you swap any foods you don't eat for the equivalent amount of a food you do – remembering that you might need to add some extra fat to things like white fish or shellfish.

Generally, vegetarian alternatives like tofu, TVP, etc. contain a few too many carbohydrates and not enough fat and protein to work perfectly on the plan. It's okay to have them for one meal every two or three days maximum if you're really struggling, but you may find your results stall a bit on those days. It's better to avoid them until you reach Maintenance if you can.

Vegetables

Most people when they try and lose weight increase the amount of vegetables they eat. Not on this plan. While two suggested meals a day do contain vegetables they are in small portions with only green and white vegetables allowed. Again, the vegetables chosen for this plan comes down to how they affect insulin levels.

The speed with which food raises insulin in the system is measured by something called the glycaemic index. To calculate this scientists feed the amount of food that contains 50 g (2 oz) of carbohydrate to a volunteer and measure what happens to their blood-sugar level. This is then compared against what happens if someone eats 50 g (2 oz) of pure glucose and the foods are given a specific number.

Any food that scores under 55 is classed as a low-GI food and pretty much all vegetables appear in this group. However, just because a vegetable has a low-GI ranking doesn't mean that it doesn't raise insulin at all. Every single food that contains a carbohydrate will raise insulin to some extent, so what you're trying to do is pick the ones that raise it least. These are the ones with the lowest numbered rankings on the GI scale. Parsnips, for example, have a rating of 52, sweet corn is 55, watercress is only 32. Once you start the 10-Day Blitz therefore, you'll be eating only green leafy veg, most other green vegetables and some white vegetables, all of which cause the lowest insulin response. Also remember the darker the vegetable the more nutrients it contains, that's why you'll find we recommend a lot of darker green vegetables like spinach, broccoli or rocket as your side dishes.

ALLOWED

Alfalfa sprouts, all green lettuce, artichokes, asparagus, aubergine, bamboo shoots, beansprouts, bok choy, broccoli, broccolini, Brussels sprouts, cauliflower, cavolo nero, celery, courgette, cucumber, edamame, fennel, green beans, green chilli peppers, green pepper, jalapenos, kale, leeks, marrow, mushrooms, okra, Padron peppers, peas, rocket, runner beans, samphire, savoy cabbage, seaweed, spinach, spring greens, spring onions, Swiss chard, watercress, white cabbage

AVOID

Any vegetables that aren't green or white – and the following that are: root vegetables like celeriac, parsnips, potatoes, radishes, swede. Vegetables that can caramelise, such as onions or shallots

Why a spiraliser is your friend

Even though you're choosing the lowest-GI vegetables, portions are still limited on this plan to ensure insulin is kept very low. This can make meals look a little bit sparse on greenery. Chopping and dicing can help make a little seem to go a long way, but if you really want to make a small piece of vegetable look like a pile of vegetables you need a spiraliser. It turns vegetables like courgette, marrow, cucumber, leek and cabbage into thin curly ribbons and you'll be amazed how much it now looks like you're about to consume.

Fruits

Fruits are not allowed at all on the 10-Day Blitz. While they are a great source of nutrients, all fruits contain carbohydrates and sugar and because of this they raise insulin too much for optimum results on this part of the plan. For these 10 days you must avoid all fruits completely. The only exceptions are avocados, which are an oddity in the fruit world as they are predominantly fat.

Herbs and spices

Eating should always be enjoyable and that wouldn't be as easy to achieve without the use of anything to pep up your meals on the plan. Herbs and spices are used in such small quantities they have a negligible influence on insulin levels and so it's okay to add any you like to any of the dishes we list. There are, however, a couple of notable flavourings that you do need to avoid during the 10-Day Blitz.

ALLOWED

Bay leaves, cayenne pepper, chilli flakes, chilli powder, Chinese 5-spice, chives, cinnamon, coriander, cumin, dill, fresh chillies, fresh horseradish, fresh wasabi, garlic, ginger, mint, mustard powder, nutmeg, oregano, paprika, parsley, pepper (of all kinds), rosemary, salt, thyme, turmeric

AVOID

Any ready-made rubs or mixes which may have sugar added

What about dressings, sauces and condiments?

Most of these are not allowed as they add sugar – for example, 17 g (0.68 oz) or a tablespoon of tomato ketchup contains 3.7 g (0.15 oz) of sugar – that's nearly a teaspoon's worth. Balsamic vinegar often has sugar added and even full-fat ready-made mayonnaise contains a sprinkling of sugar.

> ### ALLOWED
>
> Dijon mustard, lemon juice, lime juice, Tabasco, vinegars like malt, red wine and white
>
> ### AVOID
>
> Gravy, fish sauce, horseradish sauce, ketchup, mayonnaise, any mustard with added sugar, salad cream, stocks, soy sauce, tartar sauce, vinaigrette

If you don't want to eat your salads naked, we've included recipes for a homemade mayonnaise, a pesto and Zana's salad dressing on pages 106–108. Add 1–2 teaspoons of these to your lunchtime salad. Other vegetables can be cooked in a little butter or olive oil – adding a little garlic, parsley or other herbs. The cream cheese that features in many recipes also melts well and can be poured over vegetables or meat and fish. We also include recipes for a homemade horseradish sauce (see page 109) that you can add to meals.

Do I need to take any supplements?

The plan is probably more nutritious than you think – eggs, for example, contain high levels of nutrients, as do oily fish, while the B vitamins we normally associate with grain-based foods also appear in leafy greens, nuts and many animal products from eggs to red meat. But that said, any restricted food plan may result in consuming fewer nutrients than you are used to and so it may be worth considering a good-quality multivitamin or mineral supplement.

In addition, the key to keeping weight off long term is in the building of muscle, and from Zana's experience the right supplements can really aid this process. She's found that clients taking them tend to recover better and therefore have more stamina and endurance with the training allowing them to train with more intensity. This in turn means better results all round but especially in terms of developing muscle tone and keeping weight off. If you do want to take supplements, here are some to consider:

- A good-quality multivitamin and mineral.
- A high-quality omega-3 or krill oil supplement. In studies this has also been shown to boost the heart-health effects of high-fat, low-carb plans.
- A magnesium supplement, which helps release energy from cells and relax muscles helping prevent post-training soreness.
- Creatine. If you want to improve muscle tone this can help promote faster muscle growth. Creatine is essential to power the explosive stage of exercise, for example, if you sprint up a flight of stairs it's creatine that's fuelling you. Your body's stores can be used up very quickly with any intensive exercise. Supplementation helps ensure your levels are high enough that you can train consistently with maximum intensity.
- Amino acids (free form or BCAA). These are the building blocks of your entire body from skin to nails and hair – plus they repair and build muscle tissue. Normally we get amino acids from protein foods, however, supplementing with them can help recovery after training and improve muscle tone.

If you don't have a favourite brand, some suggestions can be found in Appendix 2, page 250.

WATCH THE SNEAKY SUGAR SUPPLIERS

Sugar is such a big part of our diet that often we don't even realise exactly what it's in. During this plan watch out for any of the following:

- Packaged foods. Read the labels of smoked salmon, bacon, chorizo, pancetta, etc. very carefully. Don't look at the 'pie chart' on the front, instead look at the ingredients. If you see the word sugar (or sucrose, glucose, maltose – or anything else that ends in –ose) make another choice. If you're finding it hard to find a totally sugar-free brand of items like bacon, choose one with less than 0.5 g per 100 g, the lower the better. See our suggestions on page 252.
- Bottled water with any kind of flavouring or vitamins added. Again, check the label. Most add sugar or a sweetener.
- Cough syrups, cough sweets and cold medicines. They contain sugar and will stall the plan.
- Chewing gum. Even sugar-free gum can stop results.
- Chewable or effervescent vitamins.
- Flavoured/roasted nuts. Some can contain sugar so eat your nuts plain.

Drinks

Did you know that 16 per cent of the calories from added sugar in the average adult diet come from soft drinks? Drink a small glass of cola and you could be consuming over four teaspoons of sugar, in which case you're most definitely going to trigger a spike in your insulin levels and undo all your hard work. As such the list of drinks you can consume on the plan may seem somewhat limited.

Don't go thirsty though. Not only do we commonly confuse sensations of thirst with hunger, causing us to want to eat more, fruit and vegetables normally supply us with at least 22 per cent of our water intake throughout the day and the more fruit and vegetables you normally consume the greater this percentage is likely to be. But because you're cutting back on fruit and vegetables, some people might need to drink a little bit more than normal to make up for that.

Others might find completely the opposite occurs. Breads, cereals and many processed foods often contain high levels of salt, which can increase our need for fluid. On top of this, the fibre in wholegrain carbohydrates and cereals requires liquid to push it through the intestines meaning we need a higher fluid intake. Depending on how your body reacts to the changes in your diet, you may find you want to consume less liquid.

The rule is drink when you feel you need it and, to check you're staying hydrated, look at the colour of your urine. It should be somewhere between the colour of lemon juice and light straw – anything lighter means you're drinking a bit more than you really need; anything darker says you may need a bit more fluid to function optimally. Do remember that if you're taking a vitamin supplement with lots of B vitamins your urine will look very yellow, no matter how hydrated you are!

ALLOWED

Black coffee/tea, herbal teas, green tea, hot water and coconut oil, sparkling water, still water, tea/coffee with butter, tea/coffee with coconut oil, tea/coffee with double cream (see box on page 53)

AVOID

Alcohol, bottled water with any form of sugar or sweetener, coconut milk, coconut water, fizzy drinks (including diet versions), flavoured milk drinks, juices (including vegetable juices), milk, milky coffees, nut milks, oat milk, probiotic drinks, rice milk, smoothies, soy milk, squashes and cordials, tea with milk

Why no diet drinks?

While studies on artificial sweeteners seem to indicate that the majority of them don't influence insulin levels, some like xylitol can raise things very slightly. Some sweeteners also lead to bloating in people sensitive to them, and they may give you a taste for sweet foods that make it difficult to stay focused on the plan. Finally, one new study suggests artificial sweeteners may increase how your body reacts to glucose, making you less able to control the levels in your bloodstream.[24] It's possible that when exposed to sweeteners, some gut bacteria produce substances that create a response in the body that actually makes sugar harder for us to use and more likely to be stored as fat. Because of all of this, it's best to just avoid them entirely during both the Pretox and the 10-Day Blitz.

BUTTER IN COFFEE AND TEA?

While some people can drink caffeine with no problems, others find it can trigger jittery feelings, leading to plummeting energy levels and an increased risk of sugar cravings. Adding fat – be that butter, coconut oil or a teaspoon or two of double cream to your tea or coffee – seems to help smooth out those sensations. However, it also does more than that. As you'll see when you start the plan, appetite reduces very quickly. Within a day or two you might find that you actually don't want to eat more than two meals a day. Having a fat-fuelled drink first thing can help fill the breakfast gap if that's the meal you choose to miss – it just tastes a little more satisfying than black tea or coffee. Only have one or two cups though. If you're fat-fuelling too many drinks throughout the day you can end up adding too many calories. One client of Zana's, whose results seemed to be plateauing, was unwittingly adding an extra 600 calories a day to her diet via cream in coffee. This is the equivalent of an extra meal! While the metabolic advantage does allow some element of liberty with calories, adding that many on top of your meals is likely to slow or stop results.

Chapter 3

THE 4-DAY PRETOX

Eating plans and recipes

I t's time to begin and for the next four days you're going to be following a plan focusing on low to moderately rated GI foods. The aim of Pretox is to get you used to eating fewer carbohydrates – particularly refined carbohydrates and sugary ones. You're also going to add increasing portions of fats to get used to consuming higher levels than you might normally eat. One quick note though: the Pretox is three meals a day – if, however, you normally skip breakfast, don't feel you need to suddenly start introducing it now. With all parts of our plan you should eat when you're hungry and stop when you're full. If you do want breakfast, have it. As well as preparing your body the Pretox is a good time to prepare your mind, body – and cupboards – for the days that follow.

Prepare your mind

The section on psychology (see Chapter 6) explains how your mind, habits, conditioning – and the resulting emotions from them – can determine how easy this plan is to stick to. Many of us are very emotionally attached to the food we eat. We eat not just because we are hungry but because we're happy, sad or stressed. This section will give you some exercises to help tackle these emotional prompts and the Pretox is the perfect time to get started.

We also eat simply because we're bored or because we always eat at that time of day. That can't happen on the 10-Day Blitz. You can't snack, and because the meals are very formulated, if your evenings normally revolve around deciding what to have for your evening meal, or nibbling in front of the television, you'll need to fill that gap with something fun or absorbing. We suggest that during the Pretox you come up with a whole list of ways that you can stay busy in the evening while you're on the 10-Day Blitz. It'll help if these are tasks that totally engage your brain – Helen did all her accounts and spent an entire week creating artistic masterpieces from her holiday snaps using the photo-editing programme on her computer. Or simply find things that get you out of the house where temptation can't strike. Zana used to go to the gym in the evening. Not only did it keep her busy at a time of day when she would have been likely to snack, it gave her an extra dose of motivation: high-intensity training also has an appetite-reducing effect, which most definitely nips night-time nibbling in the bud. Alternatively, this is a great time to do all those tasks round the house you've been putting off.

Prepare for the exercise plans

These four days are also the perfect time to familiarise yourself with the exercise plan, which you'll see in more detail in Chapter 5. You'll be doing it daily and it works because you do it quickly and with intensity, so you will need to be prepared. These four days are the perfect days to establish which exercises you will be able to do in the gym you use and practise them, or establish how and where to do the Home Workout if that's easier for you (moving furniture if necessary). If you are following the Home Workout you'll need to order a resistance band if you don't have one and maybe a yoga mat if you have hard floors (see Appendix 2, page 252 for store suggestions).

Prepare your cupboards

Chances are you're going to need to do some shopping for the first days of the plan. The diet is so different from the foods most of us eat that you might not have what you need in your fridge or cupboards. It's best to be prepared. The Pretox helps by integrating some of the most common ingredients so you'll have some to start you off, but it might be good to pick your first three or four days' meals and make sure you have everything you need to hand. It might also help to throw or give away – or at least lock up – any sugary treats you have in the house to reduce temptation. Remember, one of the fastest ways to weight gain is to sneak in some sugary treats while on the 10-Day Blitz.

PRETOX: THE PLAN

Follow the four days of meals as suggested. If you don't like any of the options it's okay to change ingredients around, use the food charts on pages 37–53 to help do this. While they are designed for the 10-Day Blitz, they work well on the Pretox too.

Day 1

BREAKFAST

1–2 eggs, poached, boiled or scrambled served with a quarter of an avocado and 50–60 g (2–2.2 oz) spinach

Or

150 g (5 oz) Greek yogurt and 25 g (1 oz) any nuts or seeds with 30–40 g (1.1–2.1 oz) of your favourite berries

LUNCH

100–120 g (4–4.2 oz) chicken breast served with crudités from any of your favourite vegetables dipped into 25 g (1 oz) crème fraîche mixed with chopped spring onions or guacamole (without sugar or tomatoes)

Or

100–120 g (4–4.2 oz) buffalo mozzarella cheese served with quarter of a sliced avocado and one sliced tomato. Add a little pesto (see recipe on page 107) for extra flavour if you want to

SNACK (ONLY IF YOU'RE HUNGRY)

25 g (1 oz) cheese such as Emmental or Gruyère with 25 g (1 oz) nuts

EVENING MEAL

140–180 g (5–6.4 oz) salmon steak, grilled, served with 100 g (4 oz) mashed beans or minted peas and 50–60g (2–2.2 oz) broccoli

Or

Goat's cheese and spinach frittata (see recipe on page 62) served with a green salad topped with 1 tablespoon olive oil and lemon juice

Day 2

BREAKFAST

Cold plate of one boiled egg and 30 g (1.2 oz) Emmental or halloumi cheese. Add one sliced apple and 25 g (1 oz) walnuts

Or

30 g (1.2 oz) smoked salmon served with grilled mushrooms and 30 g (1.2 oz) of your favourite cheese

LUNCH

100–120 g (4–4.2 oz) fresh salmon or mackerel fillets (grilled or pre-cooked) served on a mixed salad of spinach or rocket, spring onion and green beans. Add 25 g (1 oz) pine nuts and 1–2 tablespoons of olive oil and lemon juice

Or

100–120 g (4–4.2 oz) roast beef (pre-cooked), sliced, served with a small green salad and half an avocado sliced

SNACK (ONLY IF YOU'RE HUNGRY)

25 g (1 oz) of a hard cheese with 25 g (1 oz) nuts

EVENING MEAL

140–180 g (5–6.4 oz) pork chop, grilled – serve plain, or try rubbing with half a teaspoon of Chinese 5-spice. Serve with a stir-fry of up to 120 g (4.2 oz) green vegetables flavoured with a clove of garlic and a pinch of both ginger and chilli, topped with 25 g (1 oz) pine nuts or cashews

Or

Salmon with chilli cabbage (see recipe on page 64)

Day 3

BREAKFAST

2 eggs, scrambled with 10 g (0.4 oz) butter. Serve with quarter of an avocado

Or

150 g (5 oz) Greek yogurt and 25 g (1 oz) any nuts or seeds with 30–40 g (1.1–2.1 oz) of your favourite berries

LUNCH

Half an avocado topped with 100–120 g (4–4.2 oz) prawns (grilled or pre-cooked) mixed with one tablespoon of mayonnaise or crème fraîche. Serve with cucumber and spinach or rocket

Or

Smoked trout pâté (see recipe on page 65) served with a salad of lettuce, cucumber and spring onions

No snacks from now on

EVENING MEAL

Skewer cubes of 80–100 g (3.2–4 oz) lamb, 60–80 g (2.4–3.2 oz) halloumi and 3–4 mushrooms and grill. Serve with a quarter of an avocado mashed with 15 g (0.6 oz) cream cheese or crème fraîche

Or

140–180 g (5–6.4 oz) grilled chicken breast served with 3–4 chopped mushrooms fried in 20 g (0.8 oz) butter with a little garlic. Serve with spinach tossed with 15 g (0.6 oz) walnuts

Day 4

BREAKFAST

Omelette made with two eggs mixed with 10 g (0.4 oz) butter and 50 g (2 oz) Boursin cheese. You may add 2–3 mushrooms and a slice of Emmental cheese

Or

50–60 g (2–2.4 oz) smoked salmon with 30 g (1.2 oz) full-fat cream cheese and 15 g (0.6 oz) walnuts

LUNCH

100–120 g (4–4.2 oz) canned tuna in oil served with 50–60 g (2–2.2 oz rocket). Add 45 g (1.8 oz) mixed nuts and seeds mixed with half a chopped spring onion

Or

Pork and roasted garlic salad (see recipe on page 66)

EVENING MEAL

80–100 g (3.2–4 oz) chicken and 60–80 g (2.2–3.2 oz) chorizo, pan-fried with 50 g (2 oz) spinach or 50 g (2 oz) buttered green beans. Serve with half an avocado

Or

140–180 g (5–6.4 oz) rib-eye steak (grilled or pan fried), seasoned with black pepper, with a side of creamed spinach (see recipe on page 67)

DRINKS AND FLAVOURINGS ON THE PRETOX

It's okay to still have a splash of milk in your tea and coffee while on this part of the plan, however, do cut out all other sugary and diet sodas and squashes, fruit juices and alcohol. You can also use any extra herbs and spices to flavour your food and for these days you can also use store-bought mayonnaise or vinaigrette-based salad dressings if you want them. Do avoid balsamic vinegar and ketchups though as they are a little too high in sugar.

So that's the Pretox. By this point your body will be starting to wean off carbohydrates and sugars and your insulin level will be lowered. Fat-burning will already have started and some of you may even have lost weight. Hopefully you've got the hang of all the exercises (see Chapter 5) and are psychologically raring to go (see Chapter 6). Now it's time to get really serious and move to the 10-Day Blitz. This is where the magic really happens.

PRETOX RECIPES

Goat's cheese and spinach frittata (serves two)

6 medium eggs

Nutmeg

Salt and pepper, to taste

Olive oil for cooking

200 g (8 oz) large-leaf spinach, washed

Two spring onions, sliced

Half a green chilli, chopped and deseeded if preferred

75 g (3 oz) soft goat's cheese

1 Whisk together the eggs, a generous grating of nutmeg and salt and pepper and put to one side.

2 Warm a skillet or frying pan with a heatproof handle on a medium heat. When hot, wilt the spinach in batches for a few seconds. Pop in a colander in the sink to cool.

3 With the skillet still on the heat, warm a little olive oil and lightly fry the spring onions and the chilli until they wilt. Put in a bowl and place to one side.

4 When spinach is cool, squeeze as much liquid out of it as possible before roughly chopping.

5 Clean the pan/skillet before warming a little more olive oil on a medium heat. Once the oil starts to shimmer pour in the whisked egg mixture. Immediately add the spring onion, chilli and spinach.

6 Spoon the goat's cheese over the cooking frittata pushing it down so it becomes covered by the egg mixture. Increase the heat a little.

7 Leave to cook for five minutes so the bottom of the frittata firms, then transfer it to a medium-hot grill for a further 5–10 minutes to brown the top.

8 Remembering that the pan handle will be hot, remove from under the grill and leave to rest for 10 minutes before serving.

Salmon with chilli cabbage (serves two)

Two salmon fillets, 140–180 g (5–6.4 oz) each
1–2 large pinches of cayenne pepper
2 pinches of sea salt
Quarter of a savoy cabbage
½–1 red chilli, thinly sliced
1 clove of garlic, crushed
1 tablespoon coconut or olive oil
25 g (1 oz) pine nuts

1 Sprinkle the salmon with cayenne pepper and salt and grill for 15–20 minutes.

2 Meanwhile, boil or steam the cabbage so it's still slightly firm. Drain and cut into ribbons.

3 Heat the oil in a pan, add the garlic and chilli and fry for one minute. Add the cabbage and pine nuts and toss well for a further minute.

4 Place the cabbage on the plate and serve with the salmon on top.

Smoked trout pâté (serves one)

100–120 g (4–4.2 oz) pre-cooked, deboned, smoked trout
2 tablespoons of full-fat cream cheese
1 spring onion, finely chopped
Black pepper, to taste
Juice of half a lemon

1 Place the trout and cream cheese in a bowl and use a hand-held blender or fork to mix them together.

2 Add three-quarters of the spring onion, plenty of black pepper and the lemon juice to taste and stir well.

3 Serve sprinkled with the leftover spring onion.

Pork and roasted garlic salad (serves two)

2 pork chops about 100–120 g (4–4.2 oz) each
4 cloves of garlic
30 ml (1.2 fl oz) extra virgin olive oil
140 g (5 oz) baby spinach leaves
60 g (2.4 oz) pine nuts
Salt and pepper, to taste

1 Preheat the oven to 190°C/375°F/Gas Mark 5.

2 Place the unpeeled garlic cloves in a small roasting pan, drizzle over 15 ml (0.6 fl oz) of olive oil and toss to coat.

3 Bake the garlic for about 15 minutes until slightly charred. While it's cooking, grill the pork chops.

4 Place the garlic cloves, still in their skins in a salad bowl. Add the spinach, pine nuts and remaining olive oil. Toss well and season with salt and pepper.

5 Serve the pork chops with the salad alongside.

Creamed spinach (serves two)

100 g (4 oz) fresh spinach
50 g (2 oz) full-fat cream cheese
20 g (0.8 oz) pine nuts

1 Wash the spinach well then steam until it starts to wilt. Remove from the heat and chop finely.

2 Add a little water to a saucepan then add the cream cheese and pine nuts. Melt until smooth and combined.

3 Add the spinach and cook for a further two minutes.

Chapter 4

THE 10-DAY BLITZ

Eating plans and recipes

With the Pretox over you may already have lost some weight but now we're going to super-charge that result. For the next 10 days you're going to be following the meals on the Blitz part of the plan. You'll see there are lots of options. The plan works via very carefully calculated ratios of fat, protein and carbohydrates; if you want to get results you need to stick to these. Giving lots of alternatives makes that more likely. As the pages go on you'll also find out how to create your own meals or make changes if there is something you really don't like.

If it's normal for you to eat three meals a day, start off doing this but you'll probably find that within two to three days you only actually need two – whether that's breakfast and your evening meal, lunch and an evening meal or breakfast and lunch is up to you – although the best results come from eating breakfast and either the lunch or evening meal option. It may vary day to day. Listen to your body and your appetite and if you're not hungry don't eat. Often the more fat someone has to lose, the lower their appetite becomes.

Also, don't eat more than you need. Even though fat doesn't have a sudden impact on how full you feel, because it feels so satisfying and creamy a little can go a long way and you can easily feel that you don't want to eat any more before your plate is empty. If that starts to happen, stop eating, put the plate away and see how you feel in 20 minutes. If you're still actually hungry then eat the rest; if you don't feel like any more, don't eat any more. If you regularly find that the meals are too big for you then reduce the portions before you make them – just make sure you decrease the amounts of everything in the same proportions. For example, if you only want to eat half the cream cheese or walnuts, you should only serve half the amount of protein as well. It's not a starvation diet: eat if you're hungry, don't if you're not.

Finally, you'll see that you can choose exactly how much food you consume – for example 80–100 g (3.4–4.8 oz) of protein at lunch or 70–80 g (2.8–3.4 oz) cream cheese at your evening meal. For the best weight-loss results choose the lowest quantity of the protein food and the highest quantity of fat. If you aren't as worried about losing weight quickly and more wish to tone up or build muscle choose the higher portion of protein as well. Men may also want to eat higher levels of protein as they need slightly more per day than women do. Don't cut fat lower than suggested though. It might feel strange eating so much, but it's what's fuelling your weight loss. Skimping will not give you better results – it could even slow things down.

WHAT YOU MIGHT FEEL

It's unlikely having done the Pretox that swapping to the 10-Day Blitz will lead to side effects, however, if they do occur they aren't anything to worry about – here's what you might experience and how to handle it.

- **Low energy and dizziness**. This can occur in the days before your body realises it should be burning fat for fuel. During this time even though you could be eating 2,000 or more calories a day, because it can't find sugar your body acts as if it's being starved causing a drop in energy. Adding a little lemon juice to sparkling water or black tea can give a tiny blood-sugar jolt that changes things without spoiling the plan.

- **Nausea**. Pretox should prevent this but if it does happen halve your fat intake for 1–2 days then gradually increase it until you're consuming the recommended amounts. Swapping to lighter-tasting fats like avocado can also help until your body gets more used to things.

- **Grumpiness**, headaches and irritability. These are a side effect of sugar withdrawal and may occur during the Pretox or the first few days of the Blitz. Resist the urge to give in: this will only last for one or two days. Eating something sweet will stall the diet plan and also feed the cravings you need to break. They will pass. Just make sure you're keeping your fluids up as dehydration can make things worse.

- **Bowel changes**. If you're used to eating a diet high in fibre much of the food you eat comes out as waste. As you cut down on carbohydrates, fruit and vegetables, however, that waste will immediately reduce. You should go to the bathroom as often as normal, but expect a smaller result. However, some people do find that eating a lot of calcium-filled foods such as cheese can bind their system, leading to constipation.

If this happens, move more toward avocado or nuts in place of cheese or dairy. Or, to deal with it directly, either take a magnesium supplement which will help improve calcium absorption (which restores bowel movements to normal) or soak one teaspoon of chia seeds (see Appendix 2, page 250) in a glass of water for five minutes then drink. We don't allow them as a food on the plan as they contain a little too much carbohydrate, but a small amount will help naturally move things along if needed.

- **Bad breath**. It doesn't happen to everyone but going into ketosis can trigger bad breath. If you're worried about it, try drinking mint tea or add a drop or two of Japanese peppermint oil (see Appendix 2, page 250) to a glass of water or the tip of your tongue.

- **Feeling hungry**. It shouldn't happen at all on this plan. If you're often hungry you're probably not eating enough fat. Check your measurements carefully. Psychologically, though, it can feel strange to only eat two meals a day or smaller portions than you are used to. Remember, it's only 10 days to cut back for. Use this as a time to reassess how much you serve yourself. If you want to eat more than is recommended in the evenings, chances are it's due to boredom. Remember all those tasks we suggested you plan during the Pretox? Tick a few off the list now.

10-DAY BLITZ: THE PLAN

Day 1

BREAKFAST

40 g (1.6 oz) of smoked salmon (no added sugar). Spread with 45 g (1.8 oz) full-fat cream cheese. Roll up into cigar shapes and serve with 20–30 g (0.8–1.2 oz) of walnuts

Or

1 whole egg and one egg yolk poached or scrambled with 15 g (0.2 oz) butter served with one small whole avocado, sliced

LUNCH

80–100 g (3.2–4 oz) fresh salmon or trout fillet (ready cooked from the supermarket is perfect). Salad of two handfuls of watercress and/or rocket topped with half an avocado and sprinkled with 30–40 g (1.2–1.6 oz) pine nuts

Or

80–100 g (3.2–4 oz) halloumi cheese, sliced and grilled if possible. Two handfuls of mixed green salad, topped with 70–80 g (2.8–3.2 oz) mixed walnuts and pine nuts

EVENING MEAL

Chilli boats: 140–200 g (5–7 oz) beef mince stir-fried with some chilli or cayenne pepper in a little olive oil or butter. Serve in two large lettuce leaves with cheat's guacamole (see recipe on page 105)

Or

Pulled pork parcels (see recipe on page 93) served with one whole avocado

Day 2

BREAKFAST

1 whole egg and one yolk, scrambled. Serve with half a teaspoon of pesto (see recipe on page 107) and sprinkle with 15 g (0.6 oz) pine nuts. 45 g (1.4 oz) cream cheese

Or

Bowl of Zana's mousse (see recipe on page 89)

LUNCH

80 g (3.2 oz) buffalo mozzarella, sliced. Half an avocado sliced. Top with one serving of pesto (see recipe on page 107) or 40 g (1.6 oz) walnuts. Serve with two handfuls of rocket

Or

30 g (1.2 oz) pancetta (pan fried), chorizo or grilled streaky bacon (check all for added sugar), and 50–70 g (2–2.4 oz) prawns. Serve on a bed of rocket salad. Add 70–80 g (2.8–3.2 oz) Boursin cheese with herbs

EVENING MEAL

140–200g (5–7 oz) roast lamb or a lamb chop with the fat left on, grilled. Sauté 60–70 g (2.4–2.8 oz) spinach. Melt 60–70 g (2.2–2.4 oz) cream cheese and pour it over as a sauce. Sprinkle with 10 g (0.4 oz) pine nuts

Or

Pan-fried salmon with avocado and coriander sauce (see recipe on page 94) served with 60–70 g (2.4–2.8 oz) of green beans cooked in 10 g (0.8 oz) butter

BREAKFAST

1–2 slices streaky bacon (check for added sugar), grilled or pan-fried, serve with one whole avocado, sliced and 30 g (1.4 oz) halloumi or other cheese

Or

1 whole egg and one yolk boiled and mashed with one serving of homemade mayonnaise (see recipe on page 108) or 25–35 g (1–1.4 oz) cream cheese. Serve with 30–40 g (1.2–1.6 oz) walnuts

LUNCH

80–100 g (3.2–4 oz) of flaked mackerel, trout or salmon (grilled or ready cooked from the supermarket). Serve in 2–3 large lettuce leaves with a serving of cheat's guacamole (see recipe on page 105)

Or

80–100 g (3.2–4 oz) full-fat cottage cheese with 75–85 g (3–3.4 oz) mixed walnuts and pine nuts and 50–60 g (2–2.4 oz) sliced celery

EVENING MEAL

140–200 g (5–7 oz) rib-eye steak, pan-fried and served with broccoli cheese. Make by sautéing 60–70 g (2.4–2.8 oz) broccoli in 20 g (0.8 oz) butter. Top with a sauce of 60 g (2.4 oz) melted Boursin cheese. Add plenty of black pepper

Or

Spicy chicken wings with cheese and walnut dip (see recipe on page 95) – or replace the dip with one whole avocado. Serve with 50–60 g (2–2.4 oz) of celery

BREAKFAST

Omelette made from one whole egg and one yolk folded over 35–45 g (1.2–1.8 oz) of cream cheese. Serve with half an avocado, sliced

Or

40 g (1.6 oz) no-added sugar chorizo, (sliced and pan-fried), served with 45 g (1.8 oz) cream cheese and 20 g (0.8 oz) walnuts

LUNCH

80–100 g (3.2–4 oz) feta served on a bed of two handfuls of spinach and a few chopped mint leaves. Sprinkle with 45–55 g (1.8–2.2 oz) of walnuts and 25 g (1 oz) pine nuts

Or

50–70 g (2–2.8 oz) chopped smoked salmon, mixed with one chopped boiled egg and 40 g (1.8 oz) homemade mayonnaise (see page 108), cream cheese or crème fraîche. Two handfuls of spinach. 30–40 g (1.2 –1.6 oz) pumpkin seeds

EVENING MEAL

140–200 g (5–7 oz) salmon steak, grilled. Serve with 60–70 g (2.4–2.8 oz) courgettes, steamed or pan-fried in 10 g (0.8 oz) butter. Add a sauce of 60–70 g (2.4–2.8 oz) melted Philadelphia or Boursin

Or

Pork with creamy mushrooms (see recipe on page 96), serve with 60–70 g (2.2–2.8 oz) green beans cooked in 10–20 g (0.4–0.8 oz) butter

BREAKFAST

Zana's coconut mousse (see recipe on page 90)

Or

1 whole egg and one yolk, scrambled with 20 g (0.8 oz) of butter, 25 ml (1 fl oz) double cream and 20 g (0.8 oz) cream cheese

LUNCH

80–100 g (3.2–4 oz) tinned tuna or sardines in oil mixed with one serving of homemade mayonnaise (see recipe on page 108) or 40 g (1.6 oz) crème fraîche served in 2–3 large lettuce leaves with 30–40 g (1.2–1.6 oz) walnuts

Or

Padron peppers with chorizo (see recipe on page 97). Serve with a side of 40 g (1.6 oz) cream cheese or crème fraîche mixed with a little coriander and a tiny bit of spring onion

EVENING MEAL

140–200 g (5–7 oz) fresh tuna steak grilled or fried in 10 g (0.4 oz) olive oil. Serve with a salsa made from half a firm avocado diced, 60 g (2.4 oz) diced cucumber and a little fresh coriander and sliced green chilli. Add 25 g (1 oz) walnuts

Or

140–200 g (5–7 oz) rib-eye steak or lamb served with a portion of cheat's guacamole, or topped with pesto (see recipes on pages 105 and 107) and half an avocado. Add 60–70 g (2.4–2.8 oz) courgettes

BREAKFAST

1 soft-boiled egg served with 2–3 slices of streaky bacon to dip as soldiers. Serve with half an avocado

Or

40 g (1.6 oz) slices of smoked salmon wrapped round 35 g (1.4 oz) cream cheese. Serve with half a small sliced avocado

LUNCH

Smoked mackerel pâté (see recipe on page 98) served with 70 g (2.8 oz) of celery or cucumber cut into batons and used to scoop up the pâté. You may need to double dip. Serve with half an avocado or 10–20 g (0.4–0.8 oz) pumpkin seeds or pine nuts

Or

Chicken club: alternate slices of 40 g (1.6 oz) chicken breast with 40 g (1.6 oz) sugar-free gammon or bacon and one whole avocado. Serve on a bed of shredded iceberg lettuce or rocket

EVENING MEAL

100–160 g (4–5.7 oz) grilled salmon served with 60–70 g (2.4–2.8 oz) cauliflower topped with a sauce of 70–80 g (2.8–3.2 oz) melted Boursin and served with 40 g (1.6 oz) streaky bacon cooked until crispy, and crumbled over the top

Or

Spicy lamb meatballs with tzatziki-inspired dip (see recipe on page 99) served with 60–70 g (2.4–2.8 oz) green beans cooked in 10–20 g (0.4–0.8 oz) butter

Day 7

BREAKFAST

40 g (1.6 oz) mackerel fillet (grilled or pre-cooked) served with half an avocado and 30 g (1.2 oz) Boursin cheese with herbs

Or

Cheesy eggs (see recipe on page 91)

LUNCH

Salmon and cream chowder: Gently heat 80–100 g (3.2–4 oz) tinned wild salmon in 60–70 ml (2.2–2.8 fl oz) double cream. Season with salt and pepper. Top with 10 g (0.4 oz) crushed walnuts

Or

80–100 g (3.2–4 oz) lean roast beef (pre-cooked is fine but check for added sugar) served on a bed of two handfuls of mixed watercress and rocket and half a diced avocado or one serving of leftover tzatziki from last night. Sprinkle with 30 g (1.2 oz) pumpkin seeds

EVENING MEAL

140–200 g (5–7 oz) rib-eye steak served with creamed spinach (see recipe on page 67) or green beans with a sauce of 70–80 g (2.8–3.2 oz) melted cream cheese

Or

Seafood salad of 70–100 g (2.8–4 oz) smoked salmon and 70–100 g (2.8–4 oz) cooked prawns. Serve on a bed of 60 g (2.4 oz) cucumber ribbons and top with two tablespoons of sour cream mixed with fresh dill. Add half an avocado

Day 8

BREAKFAST

One slice of grilled streaky bacon, one egg scrambled and one whole small avocado, sliced

Or

40 g (1.6 oz) Emmental with 65 g (2.4 oz) walnuts

LUNCH

Coronation-style chicken (see recipe on page 101) with half an avocado and 60 g (2.4 oz) of cauliflower florets or cucumber batons

Or

80–100 g (3.2–4 oz) mackerel fillet (grilled or pre-cooked) served on a bed of watercress with a horseradish sauce (see recipe on page 109). Add 35–45 g (1.4–1.8 oz) walnuts

EVENING MEAL

Taco salad made from 140–200 g (5–7 oz) lean beef mince stir-fried with a little cayenne pepper. Serve on a bed of lettuce with 70 g (2.8 oz) crème fraîche or cheat's guacamole (see recipe on page 105)

Or

Spice rubbed pork chops (see recipe on page 103) with 60–70 g (2.4–2.8 oz) green beans fried in 20 g (0.8 oz) butter with 50 g (2 oz) walnuts

BREAKFAST

50 g (2 oz) CO YO yogurt topped with 15 g (0.8 oz) crushed walnuts or macadamia nuts. Add a side of 3–4 slices streaky bacon grilled to be super-crispy

Or

1 egg scrambled with 45 g (1.8 oz) full-fat cream cheese. Add 20 g (0.8 oz) mackerel fillet (grilled or pre-cooked) and 20 g (0.8 oz) pine nuts

LUNCH

80–100 g (3.2–4 oz) smoked salmon rolled around half an avocado mashed and 60 g (2.4 oz) sliced asparagus. Serve with 25 g (1 oz) walnuts

Or

Homemade burgers (see recipe on page 102) with a serving of cheat's guacamole (see recipe on page 105) and green salad

EVENING MEAL

140–200 g (5–7 oz) roast lamb or pan-fried sirloin steak with a pepper sauce (melt 70 g (2.8 oz) Boursin and add lots of freshly ground black pepper). Serve with 60–70 g (2.4–2.8 oz) spinach sautéed in 10 g (0.8 oz) butter

Or

Cheese and mushroom omelette: make with three eggs, blended with 60 g (2.4 oz) cream cheese and 30 g (1.2 oz) Emmental or other cheese and 2–3 mushrooms. Serve with two handfuls of mixed green salad with 10 g (0.8 oz) pine nuts

Day 10

BREAKFAST

Morning frittata (see recipe on page 92)

Or

40 g (1.6 oz) Brie served with 65 g (2.6 oz) walnuts

LUNCH

Soup made from 80–100 g (3.2–4 oz) diced cooked chicken. Add it and 60 g (2.4 oz) sliced mushrooms to 70 ml (2.8 fl oz) double cream and warm through. Season with lots of black pepper

Or

50 g (2 oz) fresh salmon and one boiled egg served on a bed of two handfuls of baby spinach and rocket. Add two tablespoons of homemade mayonnaise (see recipe on page 108), crème fraîche or sour cream and serve with 30 g (1.2 oz) pine nuts and walnuts

EVENING MEAL

Steak with garlic butter and streaky spinach (see recipe on page 104)

Or

140–200 g (5–7 oz) fresh trout fillet grilled. Serve with 60–70 g (2.2–2.4 oz) buttered green beans, and 35 g (1.4 oz) sour cream mixed with fresh dill and 35 g (1.4 oz) of walnuts

HOW TO MAKE YOUR OWN MEALS

If you don't like any meal on the plan there are lots of different ways to alter things. The first option is to learn how to make your own meal. Here's how to do it.

Breakfast

Have a maximum of 40 g (1.6 oz) of any food from the protein list (see pages 39–43) or 1 whole egg plus an extra yolk (when boiling cook the whole egg and just scoop out the yolk) plus a mininum of 65–75 g (2.4–3 oz) of any food from the fat list (see pages 37–9). You can mix and match as many of these as you like to create the required 65–75 g (2.4–3.2 oz) amount of fat or have one whole small avocado.

Lunch

Have 80–100 g (3.2–4 oz) of any food from our protein list plus a small green salad (small means no more than you can fit in two cupped hands) or portion of vegetables (60–70 g/ 2.4–2.8 oz) with 70–80 g (2.8–3.2 oz) of any food or mix of foods from the fat list or alternatively one whole avocado.

Evening meal

Have 140–200 g (5–7 oz) of any food from our protein list with 60–70 g (2.4–2.8 oz) of any vegetable from the list (see pages 44–6). Add at least 70–80 g (2.8–3.2 oz) of any food – or mix of foods – from the fat list or one whole avocado.

WHAT ABOUT SWAPPING OR REPEATING MEALS?

This is another great way to make the diet easier to stick to. Here are the rules:

Repeating meals is completely allowed. If you find one meal you like, or have leftovers from any recipes, feel free to eat the same thing more than once. Just note the meal-timing tip below.

Swapping meals around. You can eat breakfast meals at lunch and lunch meals for the evening meal, but evening meals can only be eaten in the evening as their protein content is too high for other points in the day. For absolute best results always make the first meal you eat one of the breakfast options – whether that be first thing or at lunchtime. It's far higher in fat than protein and really helps kick-start your body into fat-burning for the day. It's also okay to swap meals from day to day if, for example, you like the idea of a burger for lunch but can't cook on the day it falls on the plan. Just note what time of day meals were originally planned for though and eat them as per the timing rule above.

Swapping ingredients. So you don't like streaky bacon or can't bear the thought of half a courgette going off in the fridge. Not a problem, you can swap any food in a meal for a food of the same food group (for example lamb for beef or spinach for courgettes). Just check the rules as to how we classify foods on pages 37–53.

WHAT IF I'M COOKING FOR A FAMILY?

Most of the meals have the majority of their additional fat included as an extra side serving or as part of a sauce, so if you have family members not following the plan, and who might be eating carbohydrates, simply serve them the meat or fish part of the meal and leave off the fat-based sauces or add-ons. They can then add as many carbohydrates or vegetables as normal. Don't be tempted to nibble leftovers if you're cooking though – remember, the plan won't work if you add carbohydrates – yes, even a few chips off the side of the kids' plates.

Three grab-and-go lunches

We've tried to make at least one lunch every day something you can prepare the night before and take to work in a Tupperware container but if you don't have time – or don't have a fridge in your workplace – here are three lunches you can pick up from any supermarket.

- Three slices of Emmental, Gruyère or any other pre-cut cheese (check weight but they are normally 20–25 g/0.8–1 oz per slice, served with 70–80 g (2.8–3.2 oz) walnuts and a piece of cucumber, roughly 5 cm (2 inches) long
- One small ready-cooked fillet of salmon or mackerel (up to 100 g/4 oz), two handfuls of spinach, rocket or watercress. Add 80 g (3.2 oz) of walnuts, pumpkin seeds and/or pine nuts
- Two boiled eggs, one small whole avocado and two handfuls of mixed greens

CAN YOU EAT OUT ON THE PLAN?

Ideally it's best to schedule the diet on a fortnight when you don't have any food-related social engagements but if you do need to eat out, you can – in fact, it can be easier to eat out on a high-fat plan than a low-fat one as chefs love oil and butter! However, you do need to plan carefully. Indian restaurants are tricky and Chinese is very hard as both can be heavy on carbohydrates or use a lot of sugar. If you're anywhere else, try to order the following:

- A hand-sized portion of plain meat, fish or poultry served grilled or pan-fried.
- Some green vegetables with extra butter or olive oil.
- A side of avocado – or carry a packet of walnuts or macadamias in your bag and serve around 70 g (2.8 oz) to increase the fat content of the meal.
- Ask for dressings or sauces to be served on the side.

It won't always work out perfectly as chefs do like to marinate meats in blends containing sugar and often vegetables will arrive already coated with a dressing that has sugar in it but don't think of it as 'all or nothing'. It may not be perfect but if you stick as closely as possible to the menu above it won't blow things, just possibly slow them down a little. However, deciding to give in to pasta, the breadbasket and the glass or two of wine will take you out of the fat-burning ketosis stage and could even see you gain some of your lost pounds back.

WHY IS NOTHING HAPPENING – OR WHY HAS IT STOPPED?

It's very rare that the diet doesn't work, but if you haven't lost at least a few pounds by days 2 to 4 or your weight loss seems to stall at any point in the plan check one of these things:

Are you losing inches but not weight? You may have lost only a little bit of weight, but lost an inch or two around your middle. If that happens it's possible you're retaining fluid for some reason which is skewing the scales a little bit, or even better, you've gained muscle. If you haven't lost inches either though, look at the following:

Are you eating enough fat? You need at least 65 g (2.6 oz) of any of the options from the fats list at breakfast and at least 70 g (2.8 oz) at your other meals – or a whole small avocado at either meal. Remember: cutting fat too low will slow your results.

Are you eating when you're not hungry? Most people find two meals a day enough on this plan. Remember your body has switched to burning fat as its primary fuel source. If you're not hungry it is very happily consuming your body fat – when you eat it stops this and it consumes fuel from the food you just supplied. Try dropping to two meals and see what happens.

Is any sugar sneaking in? Perhaps from one of the sneaky sugar suppliers we talk about on page 50.

Are you excessively fat-fuelling your morning drinks? Remember, it's cream in your coffee, not coffee in your cream – one or two tablespoons at most and only one or two cups a day.

Are you having the breakfast option as the first meal of the day? The lunch option isn't as effective as your first meal as it has a lower fat to protein ratio and includes some greens. For best results always make a breakfast option your first meal – even if you don't eat until lunchtime.

Ninety-five per cent of the time it will be one of these things. In Zana's experience, the other 5 per cent of the time may be related to dairy consumption. Some people just don't get on with dairy. Typically, these are women over 40 who tend to carry their weight around their middle. The reason can be related to oestrogen levels. As well as being involved in fertility, oestrogen helps us retain and store fat. If levels are too high in the body this can reduce the speed with which you lose weight. High-fat dairy foods may contain some level of oestrogen. If you're absolutely certain there's no other reason why the plan might not be working for you then take out the dairy for a few days. Get your fat by mixing avocado, walnuts, macadamia and/or pine nuts rather than the dairy options like cream cheese and swap to proteins other than cheese. That may be all you need to jump-start things.

POWER-UP RESULTS EVEN FURTHER

When you get to day 8 you should have lost a significant amount of weight – but if you want to power things up a little further it is possible to supercharge the plan by doing the following for days 8 to 10.

- Cut down to two meals a day if you haven't done so already.
- Cut your protein. If you're eating lunch, reduce it down to 60 g (2.2 oz). If you're eating evening meals, halve the amount of protein you're consuming at this meal.
- Don't reduce the amount of fat you're consuming. In fact, consider increasing it to 90 g (3.6 oz) per meal, particularly at breakfast.
- Cut back on, or even lose the green vegetables completely.

WHAT TO DO WHEN THE BLITZ IS OVER

Stay focused and get ready to move on to the Maintenance Plan, but before you do don't forget to retake your measurements and compare them to the ones you took two weeks ago. At this point you should be thinking one of two things:
- Wow! That's amazing – I've lost everything I want.

- Wow! That's amazing – but I could still do with losing some more.

Whichever sounds most like you we'll explain what to do next in Chapter 7, the Maintenance Plan, that starts on page 187.

10-DAY BLITZ RECIPES

BREAKFASTS

Zana's mousse (serves one)

The eagle-eyed among you may notice this recipe doesn't quite fit the rules that see you normally eat 40 g (1.6 oz) of your protein foods at breakfast. That's not a mistake. Because this is 90 per cent protein rather than the 18–25 per cent found in meat and fish, you don't need as much to achieve the same protein intake.

10–15 g (0.4–0.6 oz) casein protein powder
65 ml (2.6 fl oz) double cream

1 Spoon the protein powder into a bowl and add one tablespoon of water. Mix it into a thick paste.

2 Now add the cream and mix so it forms a thick mousse.

3 Place in the fridge for five minutes to set further.

Zana's coconut mousse (serves one)

30 g (1.2 oz) CO YO coconut yogurt or mascarpone
10–15 g (0.4–0.6 oz) casein protein powder
35 ml (1.4 fl oz) double cream

1 Spoon the coconut yogurt into a bowl and start to add the protein powder about half a teaspoon at a time.

2 As it gets thick and difficult to mix add a tiny dash of water and a splash of cream and keep mixing. If you have any cream left at the end, add and mix well. If you want to make it thinner, add a little more water.

3 Place in the fridge for five minutes to set further.

Cheesy eggs (serves one)

1 whole egg
1 egg yolk
25 g (1 oz) butter
10 g (0.4 oz) Emmental cheese
35 g (1.4 oz) cream cheese
Fresh or dried chives, chopped
Black pepper, to taste
5–10 g (0.3–0.6 oz) pine nuts

1 Add the eggs and the butter to a microwavable dish, whisk and microwave for 45 seconds.

2 Remove and stir, add the Emmental and cream cheese.

3 Put it back in the microwave for 30 seconds. Remove and whisk again.

4 If it's not quite cooked yet, put it back in the microwave for 10 seconds.

5 Sprinkle with chives, black pepper and pine nuts before serving.

Morning frittata (serves one)

1 whole egg
1 egg yolk
45 g (1.8 oz) cream cheese
1 tablespoon fresh parsley, chopped
10 g (0.4 oz) chorizo, thinly sliced
30 g (1.2 oz) walnuts or macadamia nuts, crushed

1 Whisk the eggs, cream cheese and parsley together in a bowl.

2 Place the chorizo in a small frying pan with a heatproof handle. Fry for one minute on each side so it browns slightly.

3 Add the nuts to the chorizo, scattering them around evenly.

4 Pour the egg and cheese mixture over the nuts and chorizo slices so they are covered well. Turn to a low heat and leave for five minutes until the bottom is firm.

5 Place under the grill for 5–8 minutes until the top starts to brown.

LUNCHES AND EVENING MEALS

Pulled pork parcels (serves three or four)

4 cloves garlic, crushed

2 tablespoons butter

1 tablespoon Cajun seasoning

600 g (21 oz) boneless pork shoulder

2 lettuce leaves per person

1 Preheat the oven to 180°C/350°F/Gas Mark 4.

2 Melt the butter in a small pan and then add to the garlic. Mix well and add the Cajun seasoning.

3 Place the pork in a large roasting tin and rub with the butter mixture. Cover with foil, place in the oven for 2 hours and 30 minutes.

4 Open the foil and check whether it's 'pullable' – you should be able to flake a little off the edge with a fork prong and a sharp knife should easily go through the middle. If it's not quite 'flakeable', remove the foil and cook for a further 30–40 minutes checking it once or twice.

5 It's now time to 'pull' the pork – simply use two forks and shred it so it creates thin strips. If any bits don't pull, don't worry, just chop them up and add them to the pile.

6 Divide into three or four portions and place half of each portion inside a lettuce leaf. If there are less than four of you, you can freeze the leftover pork.

Pan-fried salmon with avocado and coriander sauce (serves two)

2 salmon fillets weighing 140–200 g (5–7 oz) each
Olive oil

For the sauce

1 large ripe avocado, chopped
100 g (4 oz) full-fat crème fraîche
Half a garlic clove, crushed
Juice of half a lime
15 g (0.6 oz) fresh coriander, finely chopped
1 large green chilli, thinly sliced
Salt and pepper, to taste

1 Brush the salmon fillets with a little olive oil and leave to rest so they reach room temperature.

2 Place the chopped avocado, crème fraîche, crushed garlic and lime juice in a mixing bowl or blender and blend until smooth. Stir in the chopped coriander and some of the sliced chilli. Season with salt and pepper. Add more lime juice if required.

3 Grill the salmon, or cook in a griddle pan for about 8 minutes until cooked through.

4 Remove and serve with lashings of sauce and some extra coriander.

Spicy chicken wings with cheese and walnut dip (serves two)

For the wings

50 ml (2 fl oz) olive oil

1 teaspoon coarse salt

2 teaspoons sweet paprika

2 teaspoons turmeric

2 teaspoons chopped fresh coriander

1 teaspoon cumin

1 teaspoon black pepper

3 cloves of garlic, coarsely chopped

12 chicken wings

For the dip

25 g (1 oz) walnuts

50 g (2 oz) Boursin or cream cheese

50 g (2 oz) sour cream

1 Mix the oil and spices to together to make a marinade. Put aside two tablespoons and put the rest in a bowl or freezer bag. Add the wings and marinate for an hour in the fridge.

2 Put the nuts in a bag and roll them with a rolling pin until they crush into small pieces. Mix them into the cheese and sour cream.

3 Place each wing under the grill and grill, turning 3–4 times for about 20–25 minutes or until the juices run clear. Baste with the set aside marinade and grill for two more minutes.

4 Serve the dip with the wings.

Pork with creamy mushrooms (serves two)

2 pork chops (around 140–200 g/5–7 oz each)

Salt and pepper, to taste

1–2 tablespoons coconut or olive oil

6 mushrooms, sliced

1 spring onion, sliced

1 clove of garlic, crushed

120 g (4.8 oz) cream cheese

1 Season the chops with a little salt and pepper.

2 Heat a little coconut oil or olive oil in a large frying pan. Sear the pork on both sides and transfer to the grill. Grill, turning regularly, until cooked through.

3 Using the same pan in which you cooked the pork, add the mushrooms, spring onion and garlic. Sauté for five minutes until the mushrooms are cooked. Season with salt and pepper.

4 Add cream cheese, stir through and add a little water to thin the sauce.

5 Serve the sauce on top of the pork.

Padron peppers with chorizo (serves two)

1–2 tablespoons olive oil
160 g (6.4 oz) chorizo, sliced
120 g (4.8 oz) Padron peppers, left whole
45 g (1.8 oz) pine nuts

1 Heat the oil in a large frying pan and place in the chorizo and peppers. Heat on a low heat for one minute until the chorizo pieces start to lightly brown.

2 Turn each piece of chorizo over and toss the peppers. Heat for about one minute, then add the pine nuts. Keep tossing well until the peppers start to blister and everything is fully covered in the chorizo oil before serving.

Smoked mackerel pâté (serves two)

100 g (4 oz) full-fat cream cheese
1 teaspoon grated fresh horseradish
Juice of half a lemon
1 tablespoon double cream
150 g (7 oz) pre-cooked smoked mackerel fillets
1 tablespoon of chives, chopped
Half a tablespoon of fresh flat leaf parsley, chopped
3 spring onions, chopped, including the green stalks
Salt and pepper, taste

1 Using an electric hand blender or food processor, blend the cream cheese, horseradish, lemon juice and double cream.

2 Reserve half a mackerel fillet and then add the rest to the mixture. Pulse it until it starts to blend in but reserves some texture.

3 Stir in most of the chopped chives, parsley and onions.

4 Season if needed. Serve with the reserved mackerel flaked on top then add the rest of the herbs and onion mixture.

Spicy lamb meatballs with tzatziki-inspired dip
(serves four)

For the tzatziki

1 cucumber

Salt

200 g (8 oz) full-fat crème fraîche

2 tablespoons chopped fresh mint

Zest from 1 unwaxed lemon

1 tablespoon lemon juice

For the meatballs

500 g (18 oz) lamb mince

1 medium egg

50 g (2 oz) toasted pine nuts

1 teaspoon ras el hanout or five-spice

½ teaspoon cayenne pepper

1 teaspoon cumin seeds, crushed

1 teaspoon coriander seeds, crushed

2 cloves garlic, crushed

4 spring onions, finely sliced

1 medium green chilli, finely chopped

1 Top and tail the cucumber then slice in half lengthways. Using a teaspoon scoop out all the seeds and discard. Coarsely grate the cucumber before spreading out on a large plate. Sprinkle over a little salt and leave while you make the meatballs.

2 Place meatball ingredients in a large bowl and mix together thoroughly with clean hands. Divide into equal quarters before shaping into evenly sized balls in the palm of your hands. At this point, divide the meatballs into four equal portions and freeze any you don't need to use right now.

3 Turn your attention back to the cucumber. Take a clean tea towel or muslin square and place the grated cucumber in the middle. Wring it out fully squeezing as much liquid out of the cucumber as possible. Place all the tzatziki ingredients in a bowl, mix well.

4 Warm a non-stick frying pan on medium heat. Add meatballs and fry for approximately 20 minutes, turning gently from time to time to ensure they are evenly cooked.

5 Serve, with the tzatziki on the side. Any leftover tzatziki can be stored in the fridge and eaten at lunch the next day.

Coronation-style chicken (serves two)

4 tablespoons crème fraîche
2 teaspoons mild curry powder
160 g (5.7 oz) cooked chicken breast, cut into cubes
Salt and pepper, to taste

1 Mix the crème fraîche and half the curry powder together. Taste and if you prefer more curry flavour, add a little more powder.

2 Add the chicken. Coat with the sauce.

3 Season well with salt and pepper and serve.

Homemade burgers

LAMB OR BEEF (MAKES FOUR BURGERS)

1 egg, beaten
½ teaspoon dried basil
½ teaspoon dried rosemary
320–400 g (11–14 oz) lamb or beef mince
Olive or coconut oil for frying

1 Beat the egg and mix it together with the herbs and mince in a large bowl using your hands.

2 Mould into four even-sized round patties. At this point freeze any you aren't going to use.

3 Heat a little olive or coconut oil in a pan and fry until cooked through.

STEAK (MAKES FOUR BURGERS)

320–400 g (11–14 oz) sirloin steak, minced by the butcher
2 spring onions, finely chopped
1 egg, beaten
4 mushrooms, finely chopped
Salt and pepper, to taste
Olive or coconut oil for searing

1 Preheat the oven to 180°C/350°F/Gas Mark 4.

2 Mix the steak, onions, egg and mushrooms together in a bowl.

3 Season with salt and pepper and divide into four even-sized rounds. At this point freeze any you aren't going to use.

4 Heat a little olive or coconut oil in a pan and sear on both sides.

5 Finish in the oven for 15 minutes.

Spice rubbed pork chops (serves two)

1 tablespoon paprika
2 teaspoons chilli powder
¾ teaspoon salt
½ teaspoon cumin
¼ teaspoon garlic powder
⅛ teaspoon black pepper
2 pork chops (140–200 g/5–7 oz) each

1 Mix all the spices together in a small bowl.

2 Rub into the pork on both sides.

3 Grill the chops, turning regularly, for 15–20 minutes or until the fat crisps and the meat is cooked through.

Steak with garlic butter and streaky spinach
(serves two)

Olive oil for cooking
240 g (8.5 oz) sirloin steak
4 slices of streaky bacon, chopped
120–140 g (4.2–5 oz) spinach
140 g (5 oz) butter, softened
2 cloves of garlic, crushed
2 tablespoons fresh parsley, chopped

1 Preheat the oven to 180°C/350°F/Gas Mark 4.

2 Heat a little olive oil in a frying pan then sear the steak on both sides. Transfer to the oven and cook – it will take 3–5 minutes to reach medium rare, 15 minutes for well done.

3 In the same frying pan, heat a little more olive oil.

4 Fry the bacon until crispy and add the spinach. Toss together until the spinach wilts.

5 Mix together the butter, garlic and parsley and melt slowly for 1–2 minutes on a low heat taking care that it doesn't burn.

6 Serve the steak topped with the sauce and the spinach salad alongside.

SAUCES AND SIDE DISHES

Cheat's guacamole (makes two servings)

1 whole ripe avocado

70 g (2.8 oz) cream cheese

1 teaspoon chopped fresh coriander

½ green chilli, finely sliced and deseeded if preferred

1 Mash all the ingredients together in a bowl. Eat quickly or the avocado will brown. If you can't eat both servings immediately add a splash of lime, this stops the avocado browning.

Zana's salad dressing (makes 10 servings)

200 g (8 oz) full-fat crème fraîche
2 peeled hardboiled eggs
1 tablespoon cider vinegar
1 clove of garlic, crushed
5 anchovy fillets
200 ml (8 fl oz) olive oil

1 Put the ingredients in a bowl and blitz with a hand blender until totally smooth.

2 Decant into an airtight bottle and keep in the fridge for up to three days.

Pesto (makes six servings)

60 g (2.4 oz) pine nuts
30 or 40 basil leaves
60 g (2.4 oz) Parmesan cheese
120 ml (4.8 fl oz) olive oil
1 or 2 cloves of garlic

1 Place all the ingredients in a food processor and process until smooth.

2 Place in an airtight jar. The mixture will keep for up to two weeks in the fridge.

Mayonnaise (makes six servings)

2 large egg yolks or three small ones
½–1 teaspoon mustard powder
15 ml (0.6 fl oz) white wine vinegar
½ teaspoon salt
234 ml (8.4 fl oz) olive oil (not extra virgin)

1 Take the eggs out of the fridge 30 to 60 minutes before you want to start making the dish. Cold ingredients can cause the mayonnaise to curdle.

2 Put the egg yolks, mustard powder, vinegar and salt in a food processor (use the stirring blade) and blend for a few seconds until mixed well.

3 Now, with the processor still running, add the oil very, very slowly but steadily. Watch carefully: the mayonnaise will start to thicken and you need to stop adding the oil when you get to the consistency that's right for you.

4 Decant into an airtight jar and seal well. The mixture will keep for up to two days if put in the fridge immediately. If you would prefer to make smaller quantities, you can do so with a hand blender. A food processor doesn't work as well for smaller quantities.

Horseradish sauce (makes three servings)

125 ml (4.2 fl oz) sour cream
2 tablespoons grated fresh horseradish
2 teaspoons Dijon mustard
½ teaspoon salt

1 Put the sour cream in a bowl and add the horseradish, mustard and salt and gently mix.

2 Store in the fridge in an airtight jar for up to three days.

Chapter 5

THE HIGH INTENSITY EXERCISE PLAN

Gym and home workouts

The point of the exercise plan is to preserve muscle mass while you lose weight or, even better, increase your levels, creating a more toned, slimmer-looking body. This means you're not going to be doing traditional forms of cardiovascular exercise like running or cycling, you will instead be doing strength-training moves that work deep into your muscle. You can do these in a gym using weight machines or at home (or anywhere else you can spare 12 minutes and have space) using your own body weight and some added resistance.

Which you choose will depend on your lifestyle. The High Intensity Gym Workout will give the best results, as the heavier the weight you can lift, the greater fat-burning and strength gains you can achieve. However, we understand not everyone can get to the gym – or at least they can't get there every single day – which is why we also have the High Intensity Home Workout, a body weight-based programme that you can do anytime anywhere. Some rules to follow though no matter what plan you're going to do.

1   Work out every single day.
2   Train with as much intensity as possible.

3   Longer is not better. Quality and intensity are what matter, not duration.

THE HIGH INTENSITY GYM WORKOUT

The idea of the gym plan is that each day you work just two selected body parts – we have three different routines to help you do this. This might sound unusual for those of you used to doing sessions or exercise classes where you work the whole body in one go but the reason for it is simple. During each of these sessions you're going to be aiming to work your muscle as hard as you possibly can and as a result recruit more muscle fibres than in a normal workout. Many people think muscle builds as you exercise. It doesn't. It only builds in the days afterwards while the muscles rest and recover. Too little recovery can reduce the results in terms of strength and muscle gains and the greatest mistake people make with training is not allowing enough recovery time. By rotating the three different body routines over the 14 days of the Pretox and 10-Day Blitz you allow each muscle group plenty of time for recovery before you work it again. The only exception to this is the abdominal plan which you do daily.

Remember, the key to this plan is intensity, which we're going to create by using heavy weights lifted at speed. To do this well you will need to do two things:

1   *Pick the right weight for you.* Every person will have a different level of strength and fitness and be able to lift a different amount. In addition, each muscle group will vary in strength – if you have an underdeveloped upper body you may find you can lift as much as ten times more weight with your legs than your arms. Whatever the body part, your aim is to lift the heaviest weight you can with intensity while maintaining good form.

So, how heavy is heavy? The right weight is one that's heavy enough so that by the time you get to the penultimate (i.e. one before last) repetition you're struggling and the last one is absolutely the final one you could do at that weight. You then reduce the weight for the next set. How much you reduce it by will depend on your strength. Use the same gauge again to make sure you're lifting the right amount. If you're not struggling on the penultimate repetition you've dropped it too low – if you can't get that many repetitions out you need to drop it a little lower. If you're new to strength training the weights might be very light at first – maybe just one bar at a time – don't worry. So long as that's the heaviest weight you personally can lift it will get you results.

2 *Moving at the right speed.* Remember, you get the greatest release of growth hormone, and also get the best workout, if you lift weights quickly and take limited rests between them. Here's how to make that happen.

   a) Lifting with speed. Every weight-lifting move has a concentric part – where you are actively lifting, pushing or pulling the weight to make it move – and an eccentric part where, in theory, you wouldn't have to do anything for the weight to return to its starting point. With most exercises the concentric part of the move is the first part and eccentric follows it. In our plan you are aiming to do the concentric part of the move as quickly and explosively as possible. Really push or pull that weight quickly with all you've got, then control it as it returns. Don't skimp on controlling the return as it ensures your muscle works hard for the whole part of the move. Aim to lift the weight in one to two seconds and return it over two to four seconds. If the weights hit the stack with a clang that's a good sign that you're not controlling the return enough. The weights should always touch but you should barely hear it. That's right, all those people around you in the gym clanging the weights noisily are actually reducing their results by doing so (not to mention damaging the machines).

b) Don't rest – at all. Not in the gap where you drop the weight down between repetitions and not between machines. This is why, despite the fact that you are only doing three exercises per body part, there are six or more possible exercises to choose from. Once you've got used to the routines, you're aiming to move as fast as you can between the different exercises. Having lots of possible exercises to choose from makes that easier to achieve in a normal gym where there may be more people than pieces of equipment. In some cases you'll notice exercises marked A and B. These work the same muscles and therefore you should pick only one of them per session. You may get some strange looks from the other exercisers as you move so quickly. In some cases you'll find you have finished your entire session while another exerciser is still on the same machine. Don't worry about it, their goals are different to yours, to achieve your goals moving quickly between machines is key.

PRACTISE ON THE PRETOX

This is an approach that takes a bit of practice, which is why you should start practising it in the Pretox section. During those four days aim to visit the gym at least three times doing one workout each day. Do all the suggested repetitions and three full sets, however, don't do this at full strength, instead use the time to familiarise yourself with the plan. Ascertain what exercises you can do at your particular gym (see our machine guide on pages 116–119 to help here) and work out what your ideal maximum weight will be. Write down that weight and how to set up the machine (what seat height etc.) so you can set things up quickly when you are there next time. Bear in mind that your maximum weight should increase as you progress and your strength increases so be prepared to add new weights after your sessions so you can keep improving and are always ready to start training at the right level. Also, use this session to get used to the rhythm of lifting explosively then returning the weight in a controlled way. Taking this lighter approach will not only get you used to the routines but also help reduce the risk of aches and pains the next day. As a rule the day after your workout you should feel that you've trained the muscle (with the maximum sensation 48 hours later) but if you can't move you may have overdone things! Taking it gently over the first three sessions helps avoid extreme post-training soreness. The day you start the 10-Day Blitz is the day you start the regime properly.

WHAT NOT TO DO

One problem with this approach is that you can fall into two traps that might reduce results: using momentum to lift the weight, as opposed to the actual muscle group you're trying to work; and sacrificing form. To ensure the best results here are the rules:

- With all exercises, keep your shoulders down. If you don't you will find your neck and trapezius (the muscle that runs in a diamond shape from your neck to mid-back) will be doing the work instead of the body part you are actually trying to tone.

- When doing upper-body moves, do not grip bars or handles too tightly. This can cause your arms, in particular your forearms, to work harder than the area you are focusing on. If possible use only your fingers for pulling movements and avoid gripping too tightly with the pushing ones.

- Focus on the muscle you are working before you start. Do this either by imagining it in your mind or feeling it while you are pushing or pulling the weight if that's possible on the machine.

- Make sure you achieve the full range of motion. Don't shorten your move in the drive for speed. Fully extend and stretch the muscle and fully contract, gently 'squeezing' the muscle with each repetition.

- Keep your form as tight as you possibly can to ensure you're working the right muscle group – but forget perfection. We pinpoint the things you really must watch out for as we describe the exercises. Avoid these and then focus on lifting the weights as hard and fast as you can.

- Never rely on momentum. You should lift the heaviest weight you can, but if you need to do it by leaning back or forward, swinging or moving parts of your body that aren't the part you're supposed to working, you're lifting too heavy a weight and need to lighten it.

THE MACHINE GUIDE

This plan includes the possible use of many different machine types. This is to maximise the chance that you can find one that's free and so keep moving quickly from one machine to the next.

If you're not used to the gym or are uncertain which machine is which, the following is a basic guide. If any of the machines in the plan are new to you ask an instructor to show you how they work. It's important that things like seat height or where the handles are located are set correctly for you to ensure you work the muscle in the right way and reduce risk of injury.

- **Chest press.** For the chest. This is a machine that you sit on. It has handles in front of you that you set at chest height and then push forward. Remember to drive the move from deep inside the chest not just with your arms and shoulders.

- **Pec deck.** For the chest. This is a machine you sit on. Depending on which type your gym has you may hold handles or position your forearms/elbows against some pads that stick outwards at chest height. Whichever you choose, your arms start out at the side and then move inwards. You feel this move in the pectoral muscles that run across your chest.

- **Cable machines.** These are usually tall machines on which you sit or stand beside. Their distinguishing feature is that instead of metal bars and handles they have long thin plastic cables hanging from them. Metal pulleys allow you to set these cables at different heights so you can pull them up or down. This means you can do a lot of different exercises on one machine. You can also adapt the moves by adding different attachments to the cables like straight bars, handles, ropes or simple round clips you can easily grasp or by lying on a bench to perform some moves. Depending on the exercise we will be using many different types of these. Really take notice of these moves. As many people aren't used to cable machines they are often more likely to be free than many of the other traditional gym machines.

- **Assisted dip bar.** For the chest, back or triceps. This is a tall machine with handles that stick out about halfway up and/or at the top. Depending on what type of machine your gym has you will either stand or kneel on a platform that supports your weight and moves up and down with you. It's good because it helps support you through moves that normally need a lot of upper-body strength, like pull-ups and tricep dips. Unusually for a weight machine the weight here is supporting you, so the heavier the weight you set the easier your move will become. It's a very effective machine but it can be tricky to use (or even get on to). If you haven't been shown how to use it do ask for advice on this one.

- **Lat pulldown**. For the back. This is normally a machine that you sit on facing the stack of weights. Above you is a long thin horizontal bar attached to the top of the machine that you reach up to grab then pull down toward you. Most machines will have pads that rest on your thighs. Hook your legs under these to hold yourself in place.

- **Seated row**. For the back. The clue is in the name here – it's a seated machine. Depending what type your gym has it may be a large machine with fixed handles that you pull towards you or a machine with a bench you sit on and place your feet in front of you. You then pull a V-shaped handle or bar toward you via a chain or cable.

- **Shoulder press**. For the shoulders. This is a machine you sit on. It has two individual handles, shoulder-width apart, at chin height. Normally you'll see people facing forward on the machine pushing the handles upwards. In one of our moves though you'll face backwards which turns it into a machine that can also work the back.

- **Rear deltoid machine**. For the shoulders. This is a machine you sit on. You'll be facing the weight stack and will have two handles in front of you. Sometimes you rest your chest on a pad, some machines don't have this option. You grasp the handles and pull them out and back in a semi-circular motion. Your arms extend out to the side as you do this. Some pec deck machines are also designed to turn into a machine that works the rear deltoids (as the back of your shoulders). You simply move the handle position as instructed on the machine to work the back of your shoulders rather than your chest.

- **Bicep curl**. For the biceps (front of your upper arm). This is a seated machine. In front of you you'll see a pad on which you rest your upper arms and elbows. In front of this are the handles that you grab and move upwards toward you.

- **Tricep extension**. For the triceps (back of your upper arm). Another seated machine with pads to rest your arms on. This time the handles in front of you start close to your shoulders and then are moved downwards away from your body.

- **Leg press**. For the thighs and glutes (bottom muscles). This is a horizontal machine that, depending which type your gym has, you lie on or sit on at an incline. Your feet will press against a large flat base at the end. On some machines you push this back and forth, in other machines the base stays still and you push yourself up and down as the seat moves. You can also use this machine to train your calves.

- **Hamstring curl**. For the hamstrings (back of thighs). There are two types of machine for this. On one you sit upright with your legs out in front of you and place your ankles on top of a padded foot bar. You push on this to curl your legs underneath you, pushing the weight downwards and towards your bottom. The other is a horizontal machine that you lie face down on. With this one you hook your feet behind the pad and curl your legs upwards toward your bottom.

- **Smith machine**: Multiple uses. These are normally found in the 'serious' weight section of the gym but they are good because you can lift heavier weights on them. They consist of a tall frame, or two thick vertical bars with a large barbell between them. Weights are normally attached to the barbell. You stand under the barbell and drive it upwards with your legs.

- **Leg extension.** For the quads (front of thighs). This is a seated machine. You hook your feet under a padded bar that sits just above your ankles and then lift this up using the muscles at the front of your thighs.

- **Rotary calf.** For the calves. This is a machine you sit on with your legs outstretched in front of you. Your feet are off the ground resting on a metal plate. You flex your ankles to move this plate downwards.

- **Seated calf raise.** For the calves. A seated machine where weighted pads rest on your knees. Start with your heel pressed towards the floor as if stretching your calf and then lift the pads by raising on to the ball of your foot.

THE RULES AT A GLANCE

That was a lot to take in, so, here are the key points you need to remember:

1 Work out every day.
2 Take it easy during your three sessions on the Pretox. Learn how to do the exercises correctly and what weight to lift. Build your strength and fitness so that on the fourth workout you are able to begin the plan properly.
3 You will be doing three sets of six repetitions per upper-body exercise and up to 20 repetitions during the leg exercises.
4 Each time, lift a weight heavy enough that you can't possibly do more than the suggested number of repetitions – then drop the weight lower for the next set.
5 Lift the weight quickly and explosively then control it back to the start. It should gently tip the stack but don't let it clang.

6 Try not to rest between sets of repetitions and move quickly from one machine to the next. If you do need a pause to catch your breath, stop for up to 10 seconds then move on.

7 Don't add extra moves – they're unnecessary.

Routine 1: chest and back

Choose any three exercises for your chest, then three for your back from the list below. Remember, exactly which exercises you do isn't as important as moving between them quickly. When possible try and complete one body part before commencing on the second and aim to alternate a pushing with a pulling motion, however, your ability to do this will depend on how busy your gym is. If your gym is very busy you can also add in the press-up move from the High Intensity Home Workout on page 154 to replace a chest exercise.

FORM TIP

Remember: during all upper-body exercises keep your wrists in line with your forearms, keep your tummy tight and always keep your shoulders down. Don't grip too tightly and never hold your breath. For best effect with all chest exercises keep chin tilted down and slightly round your shoulders forward. For best effect with all back exercises keep the chin up and pull your shoulders down and back throughout each exercise. Finally, if at any point while doing a chest exercise you feel the move too much in your shoulders, you should shorten the movement a little. Keep it focused on your chest.

Chest exercises

All chest exercises work the pectorals, the muscles along the sternum and chest.

INCLINE CHEST PRESS OR CHEST PRESS (A)

Use: Chest press

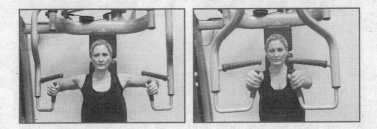

1 Adjust the seat so the handles are level with your mid-chest. Your wrists should be flat in line with your forearms not bent or forwards. Keep your abdominal muscles tight. Inhale.

2 Exhale and press the handles forward so your arms straighten, don't lock your elbows and keep your back against the seat and shoulders down throughout the move. Focus on your chest muscles as you push.

3 Inhale and bring the handles back to just in line with your chest.

4 Repeat five more times. Lower the weight, repeat six times, lower again and do your final six reps.

SEATED CABLE CHEST PRESS (B)

Use: Seated cable machine

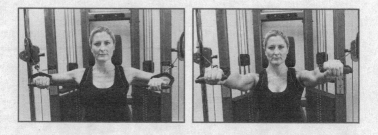

1 Sit at the machine with your back to it. Adjust the cables, bringing them to either chest or shoulder height. They will be behind you to either side. Pull them towards you so they are positioned at mid-chest. Keep your back firmly supported against the backrest, shoulders down throughout.

2 Exhale and push the handles forward, straightening your arms. Don't lock your elbows. Your lower back should stay in contact with the backrest.

3 Pause for a second, inhale, then slowly return the cables to the start position.

4 Repeat five more times. Lower the weight, repeat six times, lower again and do your final six reps.

STANDING CABLE CHEST PRESS (C)

Use: Cable machine

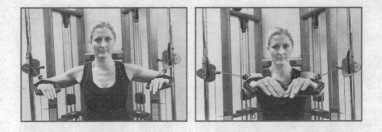

1 Set the machine so both cables are roughly chest height. Stand with your back to the machine, and hold a handle in each hand. Take a step or two forward and place one foot in front of the other, roughly hip-distance apart. Keep your stomach tight and shoulders down.

2 Exhale and push the handles straight out in front of you. As you extend your arms, bring them together so your arms are at full length, your hands meet in front of your chest. Pause for a second and return to the start.

3 Repeat five more times. Lower the weight, repeat six times, lower again and do your final six reps.

PEC FLY

Use: Pec deck

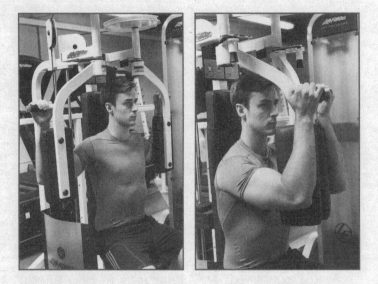

1   Sit in the machine and position the handles/pads so your upper arms are directly parallel with the floor – not angled up or down. Relax your shoulders.

2   Exhale. Press/push the handles/pads together in a wide arc with your arms bent as if you were trying to hug a tree.

3   When you get to the middle, inhale and control the handles/pads as they move back to the starting position. Keep shoulders down throughout.

4   Repeat five more times. Lower the weight, repeat six times, lower again and do your final six reps.

CABLE PULLOVER

Use: Cable machine

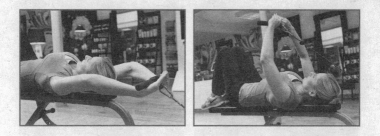

1 First attach the short bar to the machine and position the cable on the lowest attachment.

2 Place a flat bench so the top of the bench is about two feet away from the machine.

3 Lying on the bench, with your head resting at the end closest to the machine, bend your knees so your feet rest on the bench.

4 Now take hold of the short bar with both hands, so your arms are stretched out behind your head, palms facing the ceiling and hands raised very slightly towards you.

5 Inhale, bend your arms at the elbows at a 45-degreee angle then lock them tight, so there is no further movement at the elbow.

6 Keeping the arms locked but still slightly bent, focusing on your chest, push against the bar, pressing it upwards in an arc over your head. Stop once your hands and bar are slightly beyond 90 degrees, over your abdomen.

7 Return slowly to starting position.

8 Repeat five times, lower the weight, repeat six times, lower again and repeat for the last six times.

ASSISTED DIPS

Use: Assisted dip machine

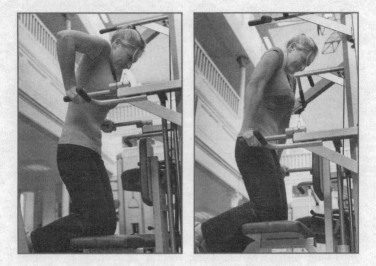

1   Stand or kneel on the platform positioning yourself so you can comfortably hold the middle grips. If the machine in your gym doesn't have grips in the middle you'll need to raise yourself up to use the higher handles.

2   Inhale and lower your body by bending your arms. Flare your elbows out to the side, round your shoulders and keep your chin down as if you were pretending to look like a gorilla. This causes the move to work into your chest muscles.

3   Drop until your hands are a little lower than shoulder level, or to the point where you feel a stretch in your chest, exhale and push back up, pressing inwards against the grips/handles until your arms straighten (but don't lock your elbows).

4   Repeat five more times. Increase the weight to add more assistance, repeat six times, increase again and do your final six reps.

Back exercises

All back exercises work the latissimus dorsi (or 'lats') along the length of your back. Great for posture and strength.

LAT PULLDOWN

Use: Lat pulldown machine

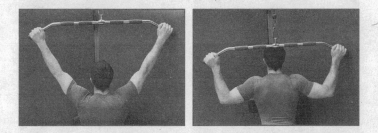

1 Check the machine has the wide bar attachment fitted. Adjust the seat height so that you must fully extend your arms to reach the bar when seated. Reach up and grab the bar close to the ends so your hands are wider than shoulder-width apart. Sit down and, if your machine has the option, hook your thighs under the pad.

2 Exhale. Keeping your chin and chest up pull the bar down behind you until it just taps the back of your head. Do not pull it down behind the head as this can encourage rounded shoulders. Focus on pulling your shoulder blades and back muscles downwards to power the move. Keep your grip light on the bar to prevent pulling only with your arms.

3 Inhale. Slowly control the bar back to the starting position. Repeat five more times. Lower the weight, repeat six times, lower again and do your final six reps.

SEATED ROW

Use: Seated row machine

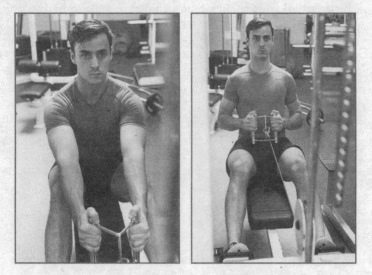

1 Sit on the seat – if your machine has a chest pad, adjust it so that the middle of your chest rests against it. Depending on the type of machine, your feet will either be on the floor (in an upright machine) or, if it's a bench-type seat, on the footrests in front of you. Keep your knees slightly bent. Reach forward to grip the handles/V-grip/bar.

2 Leaning slightly forward, keep your back straight and tummy tight. Start with your arms extended out in front of you, exhale, and pull the handles/V-grip/bar back towards you keeping your shoulders down and your elbows close to your body. Stop when the handles/V-grip/bar is as close to your ribcage as possible and your elbows are behind your body. Squeeze your shoulder blades together as you pull.

3 Inhale and control back to just before the starting position.

4 Repeat five more times. Lower the weight, repeat six times, lower again and do your final six reps.

ASSISTED PULL-UPS

Use: Assisted dip machine

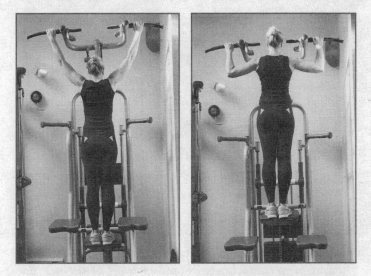

1 Climb on to the step, reach up to the top bar and kneel or stand on the pad. Remember: unlike other machines, the more weight you put on, the more support you will have and the easier the move will be.

2 Exhale. Using the bars, pull yourself up focusing on using your back muscles not your arms, lift until your head is just peeking up over the bar. Keep your chin up at all times.

3 Lower your body, then pull back up again.

4 Repeat five more times. Increase the weight (to add more assistance), repeat six times, raise the weight again and do your final six reps.

STRAIGHT ARM PULLDOWN

Use: Cable machine

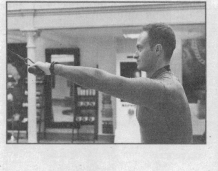 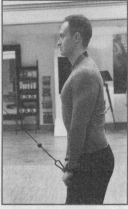

1 Attach the cable on to the highest fixing, then add a straight bar attachment. Stand in front of the machine holding the bar in both hands close to the end so your hands are wider than shoulder-width apart. Step backwards until you're in a position that lets you hold your arms straight out in front of you, slightly above shoulder height. Place your feet hip-distance apart, knees slightly bent.

2 From this position, keeping your tummy tight and your arms straight, exhale then push the bar down toward your body without swaying your hips. Stop when it touches you.

3 Inhale and return to the starting position.

4 Repeat five more times. Lower the weight, repeat six times, lower again and do your final six reps.

INVERTED BACK PRESS

Use: Shoulder press

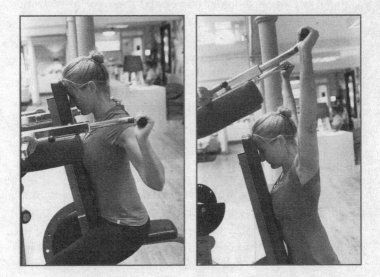

1 Normally you sit on a shoulder press facing outwards, but this time you're going to turn round and sit facing the back rest. Trainers or other exercisers may come up to you and say you're doing things wrong, but don't worry! Set the seat height so the handles are as close to being in line with your shoulders as you can comfortably position them – handles will be behind your shoulders.

2 Grab the handles, exhale and press the handles upwards while keeping your forehead pressing against the back rest. You should feel this along the length of your back.

3 Inhale and return to the starting position.

4 Repeat five more times. Lower the weight, repeat six times, lower again and do your final six reps.

Routine 2: shoulders and arms

Choose any three shoulder moves and three for arms from the following list of exercises. Whenever possible, begin with the shoulders and follow with the arms if you can. However, exactly which moves you do isn't as important as moving between them quickly. If your gym is very busy you can also add in the tricep dips, bicep curls or diamond push-up moves from the High Intensity Home Workout on pages 160–162 to work your arms.

Shoulder moves

All shoulder exercises work the deltoids, the muscles of your shoulders. If during any shoulder exercise you feel it too much in your neck you may be raising your shoulders. Keep them down and if it keeps occurring you may need to start on a lower weight to help build strength in your shoulders so your neck doesn't feel the need to help.

SHOULDER PRESS

Use: Shoulder press machine

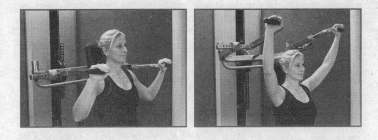

1 Sit on the machine and set the seat so your thighs are parallel to the floor and your elbows are at a 45-degree angle just below shoulder level when you grasp the handles. Keep your abdominal muscles tight and your back pressed firmly against the back rest throughout the move.

2 Exhale and push the handles directly up towards the ceiling. Stop just before your elbows lock.

3 Inhale and gently lower back to the starting position.

4 Repeat five more times. Lower the weight, repeat six times, lower again and do your final six reps.

UPRIGHT ROW

Use: Cable machine with a short bar attachment

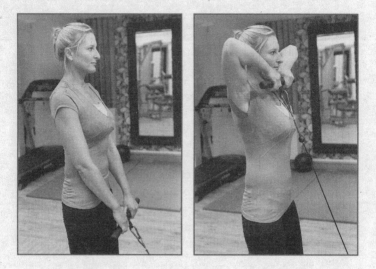

1 Attach the cable to the fixing at the bottom of the machine and attach a short straight bar attachment. Stand facing the machine, feet hip-distance apart and knees slightly bent. Hold the bar so your arms are straight with your hands holding the bar by your legs. Position your hands a little closer than shoulder-width apart, palms down so your thumbs are on top of the bar touching each other.

2 Exhale and, bending your elbows out to the side, pull the bar straight up towards your chin. Stop when your thumbs touch your chin. Keep your chin up and elbows as high as possible throughout.

3 Lower to the starting position.

4 Repeat five more times. Lower the weight, repeat six times, lower again and do your final six reps.

LATERAL RAISE

Use: Cable machine with a D-ring or handle attachment

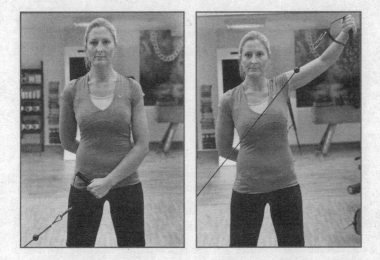

1   Position the cable at the bottom attachment on the machine and attach a small handle or a large D-ring.

2   Stand right side to the machine with feet hip-distance apart and knees slightly bent. Reach down and grab the ring with your left hand, the cable should be in front of you. Stand upright, keep your abdominal muscles tight, and bend your left arm to a 45-degree angle, fist facing inwards towards your body.

3   Place your right hand behind your back for support. With your chest upright and your arm locked tight at 45 degrees, raise your left elbow and forearm to slightly above shoulder height. Inhale and return to the start. Keep your arm at the same angle throughout.

4   Repeat five more times. Lower the weight, repeat six times, lower again, then do your final six reps. Swap sides and repeat on the other arm.

REAR DELTOID FLY (A)

Use: Rear deltoid machine or pec deck

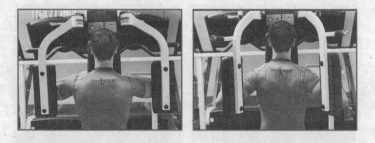

1 Sit on the seat and, if your machine has the option, rest your chest against the chest rest. Your back should be straight, not slumped forward. If you're leaning forward move your bottom forward so you're nearer the pad.

2 Grasp the handles of the rear deltoid machine with an overhand grip and draw them back in a wide arc. If using a pec deck, place your elbows on the pad and press back, squeezing your shoulder blades together.

3 Control the weight back to the starting position. Repeat five more times. Lower the weight, repeat six times, lower again and do your final six reps.

REAR DELTOID PULL (C)

Use: Cable machine with a wide bar attachment or lat pull-down machine

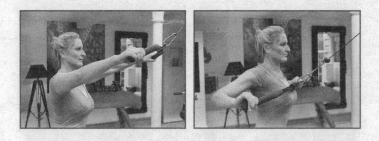

1 Stand facing the machine and adjust the cables to the highest fixing. Add the wide/long bar and hold it at the edges. Step back so you are reaching up to the bar with extended straight arms slightly higher than shoulder height. Have feet hip-distance apart and knees slightly bent.

2 Exhale and pull the bar toward your chest, flaring your elbows out to the side. Keep your shoulders down and elbows up throughout the move. Stop when the bar reaches your chest.

3 Inhale and return to the starting position. Ensure you can feel the back of your shoulders working as you return the weight.

4 Repeat five more times. Lower the weight, repeat six times, lower again and do your final six reps.

Arm moves

Bicep exercises shape and tone the front of your upper arm while tricep exercises work the muscles at the back of the arms. A good mix of both is important.

BICEP CURL (A)

Use: Bicep curl machine

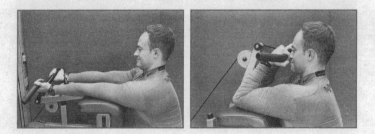

1   Sit on the machine and place your arms on top of the pad so their backs touch the surface. Adjust the seat height so that your elbows align with the moving part of the machine and the pads are under your armpit. Lean forward and grasp the handles.

2   Keeping your shoulders down and hands raised slightly towards you, exhale and bend your elbows, curl the handles toward your chest until your elbows can't bend any more.

3   Inhale and slowly lower back to the start point.

4   Repeat five more times. Lower the weight, repeat six times, lower again and do your final six reps.

CABLE CURL (B)

Use: Cable machine with a short bar attachment

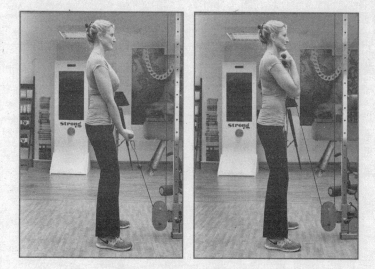

1   Stand facing the cable machine and fix the cable to the bottom attachment. Add a short bar attachment. Grab the bar so your palms face upright and move your hands until they are about shoulder-width apart. Now lift it to approximately waist height keeping arms straight, elbows tucked into your waist, hands raised slightly towards you.

2   Still keeping your elbows tucked in and the upper part of your arm completely still, exhale and curl the bar upwards until your fists touch your shoulders.

3   Inhale and lower the bar to until arms are fully extended, keeping hands curled slightly towards you at all times.

4   Repeat five more times. Lower the weight, repeat six times, lower again and do your final six reps.

TRICEP PUSHDOWN

Use: Cable machine with a straight bar attachment

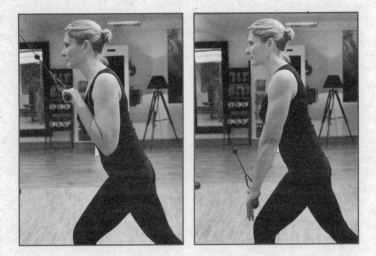

1. Stand facing the cable machine and fix the cable to the upper attachment. Add the straight bar. Take a step back so one foot is slightly in front of the other and hold the bar so your palms are facing downwards, shoulder-width apart.

2. Pull the bar down so it is at shoulder height, arms fully bent, and tuck your elbows close to your body and bend very slightly forward. Keeping your upper arms still, tummy tight and your elbows tucked in throughout the move, exhale and press the bar downwards as if trying to push past your knees. Your arms should finish straight and fully extended in front of your legs.

3. Inhale and return the bar to shoulder height.

4. Repeat five more times. Lower the weight, repeat six times, lower again and do your final six reps.

ROPE TRICEPS

Use: Cable machine with a rope attachment

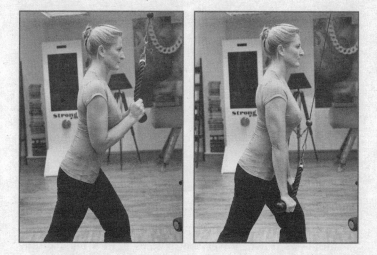

1 Stand facing the cable machine and position the cable on the upper attachment. Add the rope attachment. Take a step back so one foot is slightly in front of the other. Hold the rope so you are touching the rope part and the side of your hands butt against the large plastic ends. Pull the rope down so it is at shoulder height, arms fully bent and tuck your elbows close to your body.

2 Bending forward slightly, keep your upper arms still and your elbows tucked in throughout the move. Exhale and press the rope downwards until your arms are fully extended. Push the ends of the rope outwards towards either side of your knees. As you get closer to your legs pull the ends apart to increase activity in your triceps.

3 Inhale and return the rope to shoulder height.

4 Repeat five more times. Lower the weight, repeat six times, lower again and do your final six reps.

TRICEPS EXTENSION

Use: Tricep extension machine

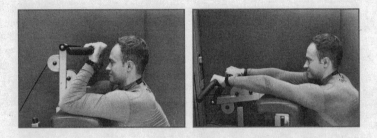

1   Sit on the machine and position your upper arms on the
    pads. Grab the handles with your palms facing away
    from you.

2   Exhale and, keeping the upper part of your arm still and
    shoulders down, lower the handles until arms are fully
    extended.

3   Inhale and return to the starting position.

4   Repeat five more times. Lower the weight, repeat six
    times, lower again and do your final six reps.

Routine 3: legs

Leg routines are divided into exercises we use to work the thighs (quadriceps or 'quads' and hamstrings) and those for the calves.

We have divided the workout into four different exercises you must do one–two options for each. Which move you choose isn't as important as moving between each one quickly. If your gym is very busy you can also add in the lunges or super-squats from the High Intensity Home Workout on pages 155–6 using dumbbells as directed to add a little extra resistance.

Choose one of the following two moves to work your quads, hamstrings – and also your glutes (the muscles in your bottom).

Note: You shouldn't feel these moves in your back or knees. If you do, adjust your foot position so your feet are further in front of you, ensuring your knees remain in line with your angle throughout the whole movement. To begin with, use a light weight or ask a training partner to help you until you are used to the movements. Always be very careful with your back and knees.

LEG PRESS

Use: Leg press machine (A)

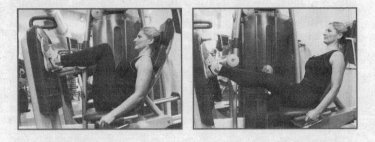

1 Sit or recline in the machine (depending which version your gym has) with your whole back against the back-rest/base. Your feet should be on the resistance pad, shoulder-distance apart, toes pointing very slightly outwards and the machine set so you can squat as low as you comfortably can.

2 Exhale while you push through your heels against the resistance plate. Keep your heels flat upon it. Straighten your legs but stop at the point just before your knees lock. You should not feel any strain on either your back or knees as you move.

3 Inhale and lower back down.

4 Repeat 19 more times. Lower the weight, repeat 20 times, lower again and do your final 20 reps.

SMITH MACHINE SQUAT

Use: Smith machine (B) (see note on page 143)

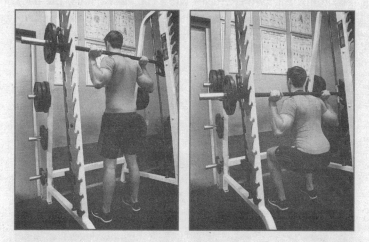

1   Stand in the middle of the machine and set the bar a few inches lower than shoulder height (to lift it easily). Position the bar at the back of your shoulders, slightly below your neck. Grip it with hands positioned slightly wider than shoulder-width apart. Lift the bar by pushing with your legs and straightening your upper body.

2   Stand with your feet shoulder-width apart, toes pointed slightly outwards. Keep your tummy tight, inhale and slowly lower your upper body by bending your knees. Keep your back upright, chest and chin up and your heels dug firmly into the ground. Lower until your thighs are parallel to the floor. Press your weight through your heels and keep your knees directly in line with your ankle and heel.

3   Exhale and push the bar upwards using your heels, legs and glutes. Stop when your legs are straight but do not lock your knees. Lower back to the starting position.

4   Repeat 19 more times. Lower the weight, repeat 20 times, lower again and do your final 20 reps.

Hamstrings

The following two exercises work the hamstrings, the back of your thigh. Strong hamstrings can help prevent some back strains and are very helpful if you're a runner. Choose one of the following.

SEATED HAMSTRING CURL (A)

Use: Seated curl machine

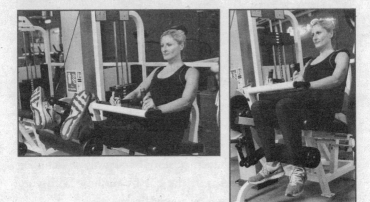

1 Sit on the machine with the top pad resting slightly above your knees. The lower half of your leg should be resting on top of the second pad, which should be positioned just below your calves. Legs should be as straight as the machine will allow. Point your toes outwards.

2 Exhale, bend your knees and curl your legs pushing the bottom pad down and under your bottom. Keep your upper body still.

3 Inhale and return to the starting position.

4 Repeat five more times. Lower the weight, repeat six times, lower again and do your final six reps.

LYING HAMSTRING CURL (B)

Use: Lying leg curl machine

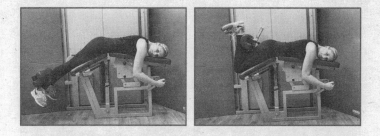

1   Lie face down on the flat, bench-like part of the machine. The leg pad should be on top of your legs just below your calf. Legs should be as straight as the machine will allow, point your toes outwards.

2   Exhale and curl your legs up behind you so the pad touches the top of your leg. Your thighs should stay in contact with the bench, don't arch your back.

3   Inhale and bring the legs back to the starting position.

4   Repeat five more times. Lower the weight, repeat six times, lower again and do your final six reps.

Quads

This next move works the quads – or the front of your thighs.

LEG EXTENSION

Use: Leg extension machine

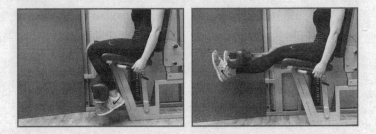

1 Sit on the machine and place your feet underneath the lower pad. It should rest just above your ankles. Keep your toes pointing slightly outwards.

2 Keeping your abdominal muscles tight, exhale and push the pad upwards by extending your legs straight.

3 Inhale and lower the pad back down as far as the machine will allow, unless you feel a strain on your knees in which case ensure you stop just before 90 degrees.

4 Repeat five more times. Lower the weight, repeat six times, lower again and do your final six reps.

Calves

If done correctly these exercises can really elongate the calf muscle. Strong calf muscles not only look good, they can help power most sports. Do one or two of the following.

CALF RAISES BY MACHINE (A)

Use: Rotary calf machine or leg press machine

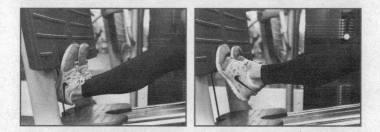

1 Sit on the machine and adjust the seat so your knees are slightly bent and your feet are parallel and flat against the foot rest. Your toes are near the top of the plate and your feet are hip-width apart.

2 Exhale, tighten the calf and push down on the plate, pressing with your toes. If using a rotary calf machine, your feet will be pointing downwards by about 45 degrees. If using a leg press, you will raise your body so your weight is on your toes. Do not move your knees as you do this.

3 Inhale and return to the start. Then lower your heels to extend your calves into a full stretch.

4 Repeat 5–7 more times. Turn your toes inwards and repeat the same movement 6–8 times, then turn your toes outwards and repeat 6–8 times.

5 Gradually increase to three sets of 12, then sets of 20.

CALF RAISES – FREESTANDING (B)

Use: A step

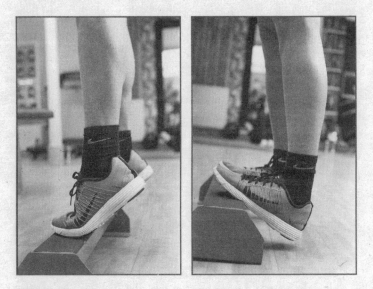

1   Stand on a step. Your heels should be slightly off the edge.

2   Holding on to a wall for support and to keep your body upright and relaxed, start with your toes pointing forwards, feet parallel and raise your heels up off the step coming as high up on to your big toe as possible. Contract your calves. Then lower heels as low to the floor as possible to a full stretch. The first time you do it do this 6 to 8 times, the next session increase to 10 to 12 and work up to 20.

3   Now turn your toes inwards and repeat the same movement 6 to 8 times, then 10 to 12 working up to 20.

4   Finally, turn your toes outwards and repeat the move 6 to 8 times, then 10 to 12 times working up to 20.

Routine 4: abs

This abs workout is done every day after your other routine and will really help shape and tone your abdominal muscles. You shouldn't feel any moves in your back. If you do, check your form is correct and if you still feel twinges, reduce the number of repetitions by a quarter or a half until your abdominal strength improves.

CRUNCHES

1 Lie on your back, knees bent, feet on the floor and hands behind your head supporting your neck. Make sure your chin is away from your chest and look up towards the ceiling throughout the exercise.

2 Tighten your tummy muscles and slowly lift your chest and back up off the floor. Look upwards as you raise your chest up towards the ceiling as high as you can.

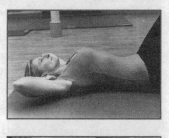

3 Lower slowly back down. Start with 10 repetitions and build up to 20.

4 Now repeat the same move but this time alternate side to side. Come up at an angle so your chest lifts toward your left knee. Return and repeat lifting your chest towards your right. Always lift your chest upwards toward the ceiling. Start with 20 repetitions, 10 to each side, alternating from right to left and build up to 40.

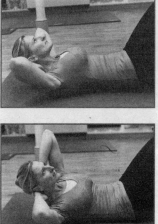

VERTICAL LEG RAISE

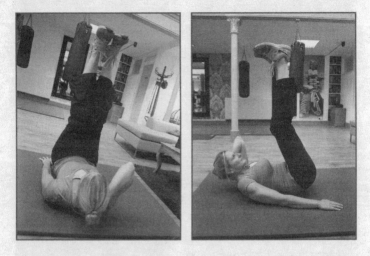

1 Lie on your back, with one arm on the floor alongside
   your body and the other behind your neck for support.
   Extend your legs up toward the ceiling. Keeping your
   knees together and slightly bent, angle your feet so the
   soles of your shoes are facing flat toward the ceiling.

2 Now raise your chest off the floor and tuck your chin on
   to your chest. Keep your hand under your neck for
   support. Contract your tummy muscles and use them to
   lift your hips off the floor and push your feet up toward
   the ceiling, as if you were trying to flatten your soles
   against it. Keep your knees bent throughout. You should
   feel this in the muscles under your navel.

3 Lower slowly and with control and repeat for 10 repetitions building up to 20.

4 Now repeat the same move but this time tilt your feet so
   your toes point towards your right shoulder. Repeat for
   10 repetitions building up to 20.

5 Finally, tilt your feet so your toes point towards your left
   shoulder. Repeat for 10 repetitions building up to 20.

WHAT ABOUT FREE WEIGHTS?

It might surprise you to see that we don't use these in the High Intensity Gym Workout. There's a good reason for this. Yes, they have an advantage over machines as they force your body to use extra stabilising muscles to balance the weight alongside the main muscle group you are focusing on, however, when lifting heavy weights with the type of intensity needed here free weights are harder to control – especially if you're lifting them up and above your head. If something goes wrong, at best you'll drop it on the floor, more worryingly you could twist a muscle at an odd angle or drop that weight on yourself, leading to injury. For the High Intensity Gym Workout plan, stick with the machines and exercises that we have listed here.

THE HIGH INTENSITY HOME WORKOUT

If you aren't a gym member or simply can't get to the gym one day, this is the plan to do. There are 11 moves in all and you need to do each of them for up to 30 seconds for the upper-body moves and one minute for the lower-body moves – use the timer function on a smartphone to keep count or use a stopwatch so you don't end up over- or under-doing things. Aim to achieve as many repetitions in that time as you possibly can. Rest for no more than 5 to 10 seconds between each move. Once you're used to all the moves the entire workout should take no more than 10–12 minutes – it might be a little slower to start with as you get used to things. We recommend you start practising during the Pretox.

Some of the moves do need either a set of dumbbells, or a resistance band to add some extra weight. If you've never used a resistance band they're actually a very underrated piece of equipment. Inexpensive to buy and easy to store, they help your muscles work harder. The shorter you make the band the harder your muscles will work. It may also help to have a yoga mat – especially if you have wooden floors, which can be tough on your knees.

The routine is designed for anyone of moderate fitness and you may find some exercises easier than others. Those used to running or cycling for example will blast through the lower-body moves but may struggle more with the upper-body ones. Those with more upper-body strength may find the opposite. During the Pretox try the moves exactly as suggested. If you find them too easy or too hard then try the modifications suggested underneath.

LUNGES. FOR THIGHS, GLUTES, CORE STRENGTH AND OVERALL STRENGTH AND FITNESS

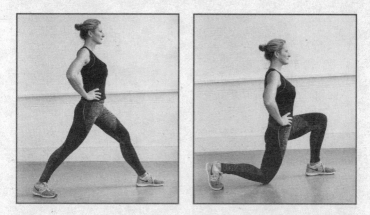

1 Stand with your feet hip-distance apart, hands on your hips or if you have dumbbells hold one in each hand and hang your arms down by your sides. Take a big step forward with your left leg.

2 Now lower your right knee toward the floor aiming to just touch the surface. Right hip, shoulder and knee should all be on the same vertical line and your left knee should be above your left ankle.

3 Push through your left heel to straighten your legs and return to the initial starting position. Quickly alternate legs, taking a large step forward with the right leg. Then lower your left knee to the floor. Repeat, alternating legs, for 60 seconds.

Modifications

Too hard? Don't use the dumbbells. Place your hands behind your head and don't drop your knee as low. Try to reach about 2.5–5 cm (1–2 inches) off the floor.

Too easy? Increase the time to two minutes without rest.

SUPER-SQUATS. FOR THIGHS, GLUTES, CORE STRENGTH AND OVERALL STRENGTH AND FITNESS

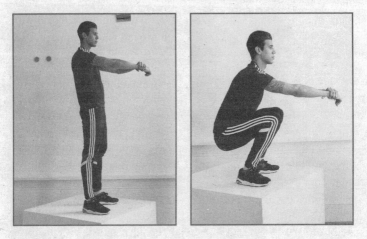

1   Stand with legs hip-width apart, toes facing slightly out.

2   Keeping your upper body straight, hold your arms in front of you, one hand taking hold of your other wrist for balance. Squat down as low as you can comfortably go pushing your hips slightly back, keeping feet firmly planted on the floor. Inhale as you go down.

3   Exhale, keeping your tummy tight, push up through your heels, and using your glutes as well as your thighs to power the move, return to the start position.

4   Repeat as many as you can for 60 seconds.

Modifications

Too hard? Place your hands behind your head or hold on to a solid structure like a door frame for support and only drop down to the point where your thighs are parallel to the floor.

Too easy? Add a dumbbell in each hand or place a resistance band under your feet with an end held in each hand and pull against this as you stand up.

PRESS-UPS. FOR STRENGTHENING AND TONING THE MUSCLES OF THE CHEST (PECTORALS) BUT ALSO WORKS THE TRICEPS AT THE BACK OF YOUR ARMS

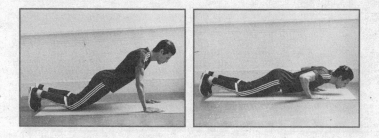

1 Get down on your hands and knees. Start with hands at shoulder level, slightly wider than shoulder-distance apart, fingers pointing forwards. Now walk your hands as far forward as you comfortably can. Keep the majority of your body weight on your hands while still maintaining your balance with knees on the floor.

2 Keeping your abdominal muscles tight, bend your elbows to lower your chest almost to the ground.

3 Press up quickly, straightening your arms to take you back to the starting position. Repeat as many as you can for 30 seconds.

Modifications

Too hard? Walk your hands back a little, returning a little closer to the original starting position of knees directly under your hips.

Too easy? Walk your feet back lifting your knees off the floor so you are in a full press-up position. And/or repeat for 60 seconds without a rest.

SEATED ROWS. FOR STRENGTHENING AND TONING THE LATISSIMUS DORSI MUSCLES IN YOUR BACK. WHEN DONE CORRECTLY THIS HELPS IMPROVE POSTURE

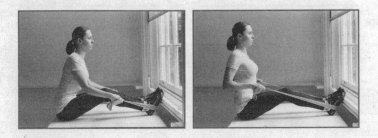

1   Sit on the floor, facing the wall, legs outstretched, knees slightly bent.

2   Hold each end of a resistance band in each hand and loop the middle around the soles of your feet. Place your feet against the wall. Your arms should be positioned so your elbows are out in front of you with a slight bend and palms facing each other. Body should be leaning forward, chin up.

3   Pull the band backwards moving your body into an upright position, chest up, shoulders down and squeezing your shoulder blades together. Bring your hands in as close to your lower rib cage as possible.

4   Return to the start position and repeat for 30 seconds.

Modifications
Too hard? Make the resistance band less tight.
Too easy? Increase the tautness of the resistance band and/ or repeat for 60 seconds without rest.

LATERAL RAISE. FOR TONING AND STRENGTHENING YOUR SHOULDERS

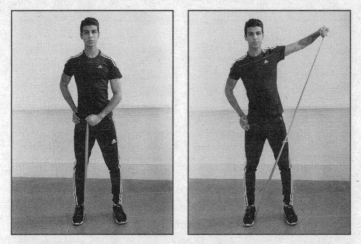

1 Standing upright hold the end of the resistance band or a dumbbell in your left hand. Place the other end of the band under your right foot.

2 With knees slightly bent, feet hip-distance apart and abdominal muscles tight, bend your left arm at a 45-degree angle and position across your lower body with your hand pointing toward the floor. Face your palm inwards towards your lower abdomen.

3 Keeping your arm locked tight in that 45-degree angle, raise your left elbow and forearm to slightly above shoulder height so your little finger is tilted upwards towards the ceiling. Then lower. Repeat for 30 seconds then swap sides.

Modifications

Too hard? Make the resistance band less tight or don't use the dumbbell.

Too easy? Increase the tautness of the resistance and/or repeat for 60 seconds without a rest.

TRICEP DIPS. FOR YOUR TRICEPS AT THE BACK OF YOUR UPPER ARM

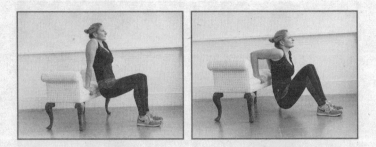

1   Sit on the edge of a bench, sturdy chair, sofa or bed, feet flat on the ground. Walk your feet forward a few steps so your knees are over your ankles, then supporting yourself with your arms, lower your hips off the surface.

2   Inhaling, dip your hips as low as you comfortably can, bending your arms at the elbows. If you start to feel strain in your shoulders that's too low for you to go, so raise up a little.

3   Straighten your arms and as you exhale push yourself quickly back up. Repeat for 30 seconds.

> *Modifications*
>
> **Too hard?** Don't drop as low until you build up your strength.
> **Too easy?** Walk until your legs are stretched out in front of you with only the back of your heels supporting you on the floor, keep your tummy tight for additional support and/or, repeat for 60 seconds.

BICEP CURLS. WORKS YOUR BICEPS, THE MUSCLES AT THE FRONT OF YOUR UPPER ARM

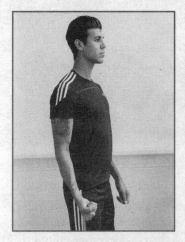 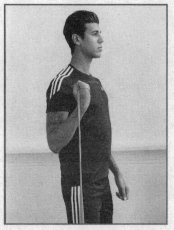

1   Stand with feet shoulder-width apart, knees slightly bent and arms by your side holding a resistance band, either in one hand and standing on the other end or, if it's long enough, stand on the middle of the band and hold one end in each hand. If you have dumbbells, hold one in either hand. Your hands should be raised slightly towards you.

2   Bend your elbows and stretch the band, or bring the dumbbells upwards toward your shoulder. Control the move with the bicep muscles in the middle of your upper arm. Do not swing back and forth.

3   Lower slowly. Repeat for 30 seconds then, if you are working one arm at a time, swap arms and work the other side.

Modifications

Too hard? Lighten the weight or make the resistance band less taut.

Too easy? Increase the tautness of the resistance and/or repeat the move for 60 seconds without rest.

DIAMOND PUSH-UP. FOR YOUR TRICEPS AT THE BACK OF THE UPPER ARM.

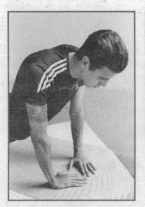 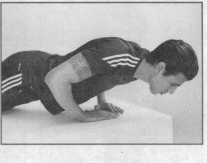

1 Get down on your hands and knees. Start with your hands at shoulder level, slightly wider than shoulder-width apart, with fingers pointing forwards. Walk your hands as far forward as you comfortably can while still maintaining your balance with knees on the floor, weight supported on your hands.

2 Keeping your abdominal muscles tight, bend your elbows to lower your chest almost to the ground.

3 Now push yourself up quickly straightening your arms to take you back to the starting position. You should feel this move in your triceps. Repeat for 30 seconds.

Modifications

Too hard? Walk your hands back a little, returning a little closer to the original starting position of knees directly under your hips.

Too easy? Walk your feet back lifting your knees off the floor so you're in a full press-up position and/or repeat for 60 seconds without rest.

CALF RAISES. TONES AND SHAPES THE CALVES

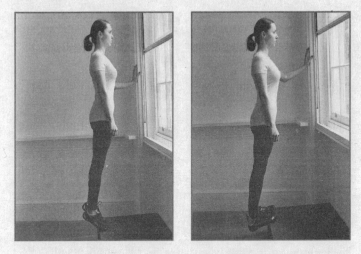

1   Stand on a step, the bottom stair or a large sturdy book.

2   Using the banister or a wall for balance, start with your toes pointing forwards and your heels overhanging the edge of the step. Raise your heels, coming as high up on to your big toe as possible. Contract your calves. Then lower heels as low as possible to a full stretch. Repeat as many times as possible for 20 seconds.

3   Now turn your toes inwards and repeat the same full movement keeping the weight on the big toe and inside of the foot for 20 seconds.

4   Finally, turn your toes outwards and repeat for 20 seconds.

Modifications

Too hard? Reduce to 10 seconds on each move until your strength increases.

Too easy? Use only one leg at a time balancing your other leg on the back of the one you're working. And/or increase to 30 seconds per leg.

CRUNCHES

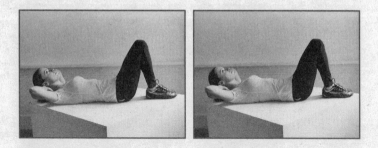

1 Lie on your back, knees bent, feet on the floor and hands behind your head supporting your neck. Make sure your chin is away from your chest and look up towards the ceiling throughout the exercise.

2 Tighten your tummy muscles and slowly lift your chest and back up off the floor. Look upwards as you raise your chest up towards the ceiling as high as you can.

3 Lower slowly back down. Start with 10 repetitions and build up to 20.

4 Now repeat the same move but this time alternate side to side. Come up at an angle so your chest lifts toward your left knee. Return and repeat lifting your chest towards your right. Always lift your chest upwards toward the ceiling. Start with 20 repetitions, 10 to each side, alternating from right to left and build up to 40.

Modifications

Too hard? Reduce repetitions on each move to 10 until your strength increases.
Too easy? Increase up to 40 repetitions.

VERTICAL LEG RAISE

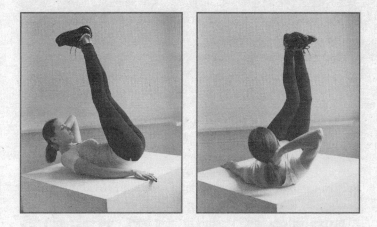

1 Lie on your back, with one arm on the floor alongside your body and the other behind your neck for support. Extend your legs towards the ceiling. Keeping your knees together and slightly bent, angle your feet so the soles of your shoes are facing flat toward the ceiling.

2 Raise your chest off the floor and tuck your chin on to your chest. Keep your hand under your neck for support. Contract your tummy muscles and use them to lift your hips off the floor and push your feet up toward the ceiling, as if you were trying to flatten your soles against it. Keep your knees bent throughout. You should feel this in the muscles under your navel.

3 Lower slowly and with control and repeat for 10 repetitions building up to 20.

4 Now repeat the same move but this time tilt your feet so your toes point towards your right shoulder. Repeat for 10 repetitions building up to 20.

5 Finally, tilt your feet so your toes point towards your left shoulder. Repeat for 10 repetitions building up to 20.

> *Modifications*
>
> **Too hard?** Reduce to 10 repetitions on each move until your strength increases.
>
> **Too easy?** Increase up to 40 repetitions.

COMMON QUESTIONS ANSWERED

When to eat and exercise

Part of the reason for this style of training is to allow for the maximum release of natural growth hormone, which seems to target belly fat and pushes protein back into your muscles. This release peaks two hours after exercise but if you eat you prevent this. For best results avoid food for at least one hour before, and ideally two hours after, your workout. If you have no choice though, don't use your food timing as an excuse not to work out. Any workout increases oxygen uptake, increases the heart rate and drives circulation through your body and the combination of all of that will still improve muscle tone. You just lose the added boost of hGh.

Do I really not need to do anything else?

No – and if you're working as hard as you possibly can you really shouldn't be able to do anything else! If you feel like you can go run for half an hour or lift another three sets you need to up the intensity a little bit more for maximum results.

Can I add cardio?

Cardio simply means the heart. With this style of training you are without question going to be working the heart and lungs, so it is cardio. That said, many of us enjoy other forms of cardiovascular exercise and if you're a keen runner, swimmer or cyclist the idea of dropping your normal routine for two weeks might seem completely insane. If you're used to spending an hour or more exercising it can seem somewhat implausible that a 10–15-minute workout will give you anywhere near the same results as, say, an hour-long run.

In this case we ask 'Why are you exercising?' If the answer is to power up weight loss, fitness or fat-burning then trust us, you're not going to get any better results by doing it. You may even slow down the result by overtraining which can a) cause muscle loss and therefore reduce the amount of calories your body burns each day and b) cause unnecessary fatigue, reducing the intensity at which you can train and therefore get results with your weights.

If, however, you do your chosen cardio training to clear your head, help you think or because it's something you truly love, then abstain for the first six days while you get used to the workouts – you might find the sessions give you what you need. After this it's okay to add your favourite cardio if you really need to but try to keep sessions to less than 20 minutes.

Don't forget to breathe

You've probably worked this out generally in life but for some reason when we start to work with weights or do toning exercises we often forget. You need oxygen to allow the combustion (burning of fuel) to occur that gives you the energy to train. If you don't breathe, at best you will get light-headed, or give yourself a mild headache, at worst you'll increase your blood pressure.

Inhale as you position yourself, exhale on the effort and then inhale as you return.

Breathing correctly also helps you relax. Ideally, when doing any kind of strength move you should always aim to relax every muscle except the one you're training and often your abdominals which are tightened to help support your back while you move. If you're clenching your teeth, straining your neck muscles or tensing your feet as you move you're actually using energy working those muscles that would be better used by the ones you're actually trying to tone.

What happens when I'm tired?

A bad night's sleep, too much work, even the transitional sensations of fatigue that can occur before your body properly starts burning fat for fuel can mean that some days you simply aren't going to want to work out as hard as this plan demands. If you genuinely can't face it, rather than just making excuses, do your workout, but go lighter. Still focus on speed, explosiveness and intensity but drop the weight down one or two bars. Next workout aim to be raring to go again, cheating on your sessions is only cheating your results.

What about warming up and cooling down?

You'll notice we don't suggest you do a warm-up before your training programme, which might seem strange. It's okay because you're using weight machines on the plan. When using these you're normally locked in a stable position and your body moves in a very steady, focused line so the muscles warm up as you train. It's also now proven to be a myth that you should stretch before you work out. In studies it's been shown this actually reduces the amount of power a muscle has and that's definitely not something you want to be doing on this plan.[25, 26] In terms of cooling down, that's one of the benefits of the daily abdominal workout. It not only tones your stomach it also acts as a natural cooldown.

Is there anyone who shouldn't do the workouts?

If you've never exercised before or have long-term health problems like heart disease, asthma, back pain, etc. then you should ask advice from your GP before you start any type of exercise. You must also stop immediately on either plan if you feel light-headed, get unusually breathless or have chest pains. Also don't do any individual moves if you find they aggravate existing injuries or joint problems.

That's the end of the workout section. After 14 days of doing it you should be feeling stronger, fitter and more energised. Depending on how much fat you've lost round your middle you might even have started to notice some muscle definition around your abs. Keep up the plan and these things will only improve even further. We'll tell you how to adapt the workouts slightly when you start the Maintenance Plan but really do keep them up – it will help you keep the weight off. Hopefully this is far more appealing now you've seen that getting fitter doesn't need to take forever and realised how easy it can be to make it part of your life.

Chapter 6

CHANGING YOUR BLUEPRINT

Finding a new mindset

It might sound strange to start talking about the mind in a book about the body, but this book isn't only about losing weight, it's also about keeping it off. If your brain isn't on board with what you're trying to achieve it's going to be harder to get, and keep, the body you want. After all, our thoughts control our actions. This section helps you change your thoughts so they support your goals, not sabotage them.

Before they meet her, many of Zana's clients have found themselves on and off diets for years, frequently losing as much as 14 lb (two dress sizes) in as little as two to three weeks, only to find their success is very short-lived. The draw of a relaxed social drink or a meal out with friends gnaws at their willpower and determination. Soon, feeling fed-up with what they consider an unfair restrictive lifestyle, they give up and return to 'normal' eating. Unfortunately this 'normal' includes snacking when not hungry and the not-so-occasional sugar-driven treat! It's not rocket science: the weight returns, and, for reasons we mentioned earlier in this book, frequently with a little more on top.

Perhaps you have had a similar experience in your own life. Maybe you have never been able to believe that you will reach your goals and find it difficult to picture yourself achieving them. You may have felt disappointed even if you have lost weight, believing that it will never be quite enough. For some of you, it may feel that you are missing out on enjoyment in life for no good reason when following a diet plan, and this frustration can lead to overeating.

But changing your mindset can eliminate that state of helplessness and break the cycle of yo-yo dieting. Suddenly, you'll be able to see your end goal just ahead of you and be fuelled by excitement and determination to succeed. You'll approach daily training with a greater intensity and a deeper focus and be able to stick to the diet plan with enthusiasm and determination. Perhaps most importantly of all, you will be able to maintain your results long after you have finished the plan.

So how do you reach this new mindset? How can you avoid giving up on the plan and falling back into old habits?

A QUICK GUIDE TO THINKING

Our mind is divided into two parts – the conscious and unconscious. The conscious mind is where thoughts you're aware of are generated – for example, 'I want to lose half a stone' or 'I want to get fitter'. If the conscious mind controlled all our actions life would always go according to plan. You'd decide to shape up, you'd fill the fridge with the right foods, you'd go to the gym every day, the fat would come off and it would stay gone because you'd act naturally in the way that made that happen. But anyone who's quit their diet or exercise plan within the first week because they missed 'normal' eating, just found it 'impossible' to stick with, or, alternatively, who stuck with a plan and achieved great results only to find themselves almost compelled to eat the wrong foods again as soon as they finished, knows that doesn't always happen. The reason for this is that whenever your mind has a conscious thought, the unconscious mind steps in to decide whether to help make that happen.

Up to 98 per cent of our actions are driven by the unconscious mind. A huge collection of feelings, thoughts, urges and memories, the unconscious has a very strong opinion of who you are as a person – how successful you should be, how popular, how wealthy – and even how you should look. All of these things are stored in your unconscious as a kind of blueprint of what it sees as the real you. When you decide to do something the unconscious brain looks at the behaviour and sees how it fits into your blueprint. If it thinks it's a match, whatever you're trying to do is easy. If there's a mismatch and what you are trying to do goes against this picture, change becomes more of an uphill battle. This happens in every part of your life – relationships, finances, career – but as this is a book about changing shape, let's explain that more clearly in terms of how it relates to weight control.

First let's look at what happens if you gain weight. If your mind thinks you should be a size 10 or have a six pack and you look in the mirror one day and it sees you're larger than it thinks you should be, it's confused. The image it's seeing doesn't match the image it has of the 'real you' and as such it's compelled to change things. All of a sudden you don't feel like eating sweets, you start to feel a bit sick if you eat too large a portion and try and sit on the sofa after coming home from work rather than doing something more active and you'll feel like you've got ants in your pants.

Conversely, let's see what happens in the same situation if your unconscious thinks you should be bigger. Then the pounds you're putting on match its image – it's happy and relaxed. It's not bothered about triggering you to lose them. Its picture of you and the outside world match its 'reality'.

At this point, however, you, as in your conscious mind, might have other ideas. The conscious you wants to be trimmer so you start to cut back, resist all the temptation to cheat, increase your exercise and lose all the weight you need. Finally, you look in the mirror and see a trim tummy and toned legs reflected back at you. Unfortunately, if the unconscious part of your mind thinks that you should be bigger, it will now be confused. It thinks 'That's not me, let's start gaining again' and it will send out all the signals and messages it can to help ensure that happens.

The problem is, if you've spent years struggling with your weight there's a very good chance that your unconscious mind is *not* set up to think of you as a size 10 or with a six pack, as otherwise it would have stepped in by now. For some reason your unconscious mind thinks you should be bigger. Where these thoughts come from we often don't know and can't pinpoint without a lot of analysis or hypnotherapy – it could be as simple as your little brother telling you that you were fat at the age of ten – now you're still here at 35 or 45 unconsciously thinking 'Yes, yes I am'. And if that's what the unconscious part of your mind truly believes, while losing weight or keeping it off isn't impossible (you can't deny basic biology) it will be harder mentally. The little gremlin on your shoulder that tells you to 'go on just have a piece of toast' or 'come on, let's go to the pub today and hit the gym tomorrow' speaks a little bit louder.

This might all sound a bit hopeless but actually it's not. In order to change something, you have to understand what's going wrong. Now that you understand the basics of how your unconscious mind works, a few simple steps can convince it to take a new direction now. A direction that helps support your weight-loss goals.

Step one: create a new blueprint

You don't need to know what beliefs the unconscious mind holds to change them. The mind is highly susceptible to adopting new beliefs without worrying about the old ones.

All it wants to do is give you what it thinks you want – give it a clear picture of that and the unconscious will capture it, retain it and work towards it. Sometimes this can happen quickly, sometimes you need to keep delivering the message over and over again for it to be adopted. Because of this, the earlier you can start the mind exercises in this section, the better – at the very least begin during the Pretox so you're ready to switch on the full power of your mind during the 10-Day Blitz and Maintenance Plan.

To reprogramme your unconscious you're going to use visualisation – a technique where you conjure up images in your head. We do this because the unconscious, while it may understand words, doesn't necessarily respond to them. What it needs to motivate it are pictures and symbols that give the words some extra depth. For example, if you think 'I want to be in shape' your unconscious might hear your wish but it means very little to it if it doesn't experience either the sight of the shape you mean or the feeling of achievement and pride you'll get when you have it.

Interestingly, when psychologists examine successful people and top CEOs they have found that one thing they have in common is that when they come up with a new idea they actually see a clear outcome in their mind for what they want to achieve. The rest of us may not find it quite so easy to imagine such a clear vision without a little training, so we're going to teach you how it's done.

Question one: what are you actually trying to achieve?

Zana has found that a client with a really clear outcome of what they want to achieve has greater success than one with a more nebulous goal, both in terms of the amount of fat they lose and the speed at which they lose it. She's not the only person to notice. When researchers at Michigan State University looked at women losing weight after pregnancy they found the number one predictor of success was having what the researchers called an 'I can' mentality. If women believed they could lose weight, they found solutions to all the things stopping them, and they achieved their aims.[27]

Why is simple. Your mind works cybernetically. It was the military that came up with a device called a cybernetic missile. These were missiles that could be programmed to hit a target miles and miles away from their launch site. Once the target was programmed in, the missiles did everything they needed to reach it. They went under bridges, over rooftops, around mountains, whatever it took. Your mind works in exactly the same way: give it a clear, precise goal to aim for and it will move mountains to get you there.

You need to know exactly what you want to achieve, partly so your brain can start doing this and partly so it knows when to stop. There is no end if the goal is simply to 'lose weight'. Even if you decide you're happy with losing 3.2 kg (7 lb), fitting into a size 12 or getting a six pack, without that as its clear outcome your unconscious doesn't know when it has achieved its aim. Its goal after all is simply to lose weight. When you stop losing weight it doesn't know you're happy, it thinks its failed. This can instil the idea in your unconscious that you are failing – and guess what? It will happily drive you towards this version of you. The first step in any change therefore is determining your exact goal so your brain can fix on its target and recognise this as the new you once you arrive. To do this ask yourself the following. Having achieved your outcome:

- What clothing size are you?
- How many centimetres or inches have you lost and from where?
- What parts of your body are sculpted, toned, smaller or firmer?

- These are better questions than fixing on a weight, but if you really do want to work to a number ask, how many kilos or pounds have you lost?
- How do you feel when you look in the mirror?
- How long did this take you?

Note that all the questions are phrased as if you have already achieved your goal – that's because the brain is so literal. If you say 'I want to be a size 10' or 'I want that six pack' the brain thinks the wanting is your goal, not the size 10 or awesome abs. Plan the outcome as if it's already happened.

The more precise and definite you can be the better. Don't be limited by past results – just because you haven't had this figure or physique since you were 21, or perhaps ever, doesn't mean it's not feasible now. Also, absolutely avoid using any kind of negative phrase. The unconscious mind does not understand the concept of negatives. Think of the instruction 'Do not think of a pink elephant' – to even consider not thinking of one, you have to picture one in your mind, then try and delete it, which is virtually impossible. Your mind works the same way with every request. If you tell your brain 'I don't want to be fat' it has to picture you being fat and it can't simply delete this, all your unconscious hears is 'I want to be fat' and behold, the doughnut cravings begin. Whenever you're setting a goal ensure it is couched in positive terms – think 'I am slim', rather than 'I don't want to be fat' or 'I have a flat tummy or great abs' rather than 'I don't want to have these rolls of fat'.

Question two: was there ever a point in your adult life that you were a shape you really liked even if you didn't realise it until afterwards?

If the answer to this is yes, do you have a picture of yourself at that point in time? If you do, go and get it, and look at it for as long as it takes to get a really clear picture in your mind.

Place it somewhere you will see it regularly, such as on the bathroom mirror, then move to Step B, below.

If you don't have a physical picture, then you're going to need to try and create a mental one by recalling as much detail about that time as you possibly can. Get a piece of paper and write down as many details as possible.

- What did your body look like or what dress size were you?
- What did you look like? Not just in terms of your body shape, but your hair, your make-up, if you can think of a perfume or aftershave you wore try and remember the scent.
- What were you wearing? Can you remember a favourite outfit?
- Who was around you? Think of a best friend or partner.
- Where did you live, what music did you listen to, what did you do for fun?

Really try and recapture everything you can about that time when you were happy and body confident and use it to create a mental image of your body shape that you can clearly picture in your mind. Now, move to Step B.

Step B: Whether you're using a photograph or a memory, it's now time to embellish it. You see, nothing in our head is actually real – if you ask two people involved in the same incident what happened both of them will recall it in very different ways and both will insist their version is the one that's correct. As such, you're going to picture the absolute best version of your memory above – and, you're going to do it so well that your mind is going to think that's the true you.

So imagine you were Photoshopping the picture or memory to be perfect. Maybe, even though you were happy, your tummy was a little bigger than you'd like it to be now, so shrink that in your head. If you were a size 12 then but you've always dreamed of being a 10, tell yourself that at that point you *were* a 10. If you liked the clothes you're wearing but hate your hair, change it so you look amazing in your mind. Create the absolute best image in your head that you can. That's what you're going to use when you start to visualise.

This is all fine for those who have a memory or photo to work from, but what if you've never truly been in a shape you like? Maybe you've been out of shape since childhood. Well, the only difference between having no recollection of being in shape and having one is having the memory. So, create one. It's proven that you can absolutely convince your unconscious with a completely fictional image. When researchers have asked people to visualise a true image and then visualise a fake one, exactly the same parts of the brain light up: if you imagine it hard enough your brain doesn't know if an image is real or fake, it just knows to act upon it.

To prove this let's talk about the 'little finger' experiment.[28] In this trial experts at the US's Cleveland Clinic asked two groups of people to imagine doing some arm exercises, one working their little finger, one working their elbow. When they measured how much the muscles in each group had grown, they found they'd increased their little finger strength by 35 per cent and their elbow strength by 13.5 per cent. Remember, they hadn't actually physically trained these muscles just imagined they had, but their mind thought they had put the work in and it rewarded them accordingly.

Now, you might want more than a strong little finger, but you can still use your imagination to help you achieve it. Conjure up in your head the version of you that you want to be. Don't think how feasible it is, or what you might have to do to achieve it, just draw yourself a mental picture. If you're finding it hard, then use the following suggestions to focus you.

- What do you really want? What does your new body look like?
- Really fine-tune the image – does it have a flatter tummy? Or six-pack abs?

- Do you have arms that are toned and slim, or stronger, firmer biceps?
- Legs that are strong and powerful? Or just thighs that don't jiggle?

You can use photos from magazines to help inspire you but remember you're not trying to turn into someone else, just create the best version of you that you can be.

See yourself standing on the scales, or trying on clothes – what do the numbers say? Really etch them into the picture.

What is 'new you' wearing? Maybe there's a type of dress or suit you've always wanted to wear, or something you've seen in the shops that you wish you could buy but it just wouldn't suit you right now. See yourself in it.

When is this going to happen by? Give your body a clear timeline – see yourself standing next to a calendar with the date on.

When you're happy with it, that's the image you're going to use in your visualisation.

Question three: are you a visual person?

Some of you will have found the 'new you' exercise really easy, others may have struggled a little more, That's because not all of us find it easy to think visually. To test yourself again, try this. Close your eyes and imagine the front of your house. How many details can you see?

If you can see everything, the shape, the windows, the folds of the curtains inside, even the chipped bits of paint on the windowsill, you're a highly visual person – this makes the visualisation exercises we've just tried a lot easier. If, however, all you can see is the shape of your house, the colour and a vague idea of where the windows are you're probably more words or feelings orientated. This is incredibly common in the general population, and even more so in those who struggle with their weight. For starters, visually led people tend to notice they are gaining weight more quickly and be motivated to change by what they see in the mirror, which often means they address things faster. Those who are more feelings orientated may wait until it's starting to upset them and have a bit more work to do. On top of this, being governed by feelings often comes hand in hand with associating food with emotions – which commonly triggers overeating and weight gain.

If you aren't a visual person, it doesn't mean that visualisation doesn't work for you – just that it might be a bit harder to create a clear image in your mind. Exercising your visualisation 'muscles' helps make this easier to do so try this short exercise daily.

Place one or two objects on a table, look at them for a minute and then close your eyes for 30 seconds. Try and picture exactly what that table looks like. Don't just remember what's on it, really try and see it in your head. See where things are and exactly how far apart from each other. Look at the light and the shade and where they fall. Identify exactly what colours things are, what typeface any lettering is in. Really try and call up every detail. Spend two to three minutes every day practising this and you'll dramatically strengthen your visual skills and your visualisation result.

WHERE AND WHEN TO VISUALISE

You can do these visualisations anytime and anywhere your mind is quiet. Many of us think that for techniques like this to work we must sit cross-legged with eyes closed. It's not true – the brain can take on information in any position so long as your mind is relaxed and not batting around hundreds of other thoughts.

Whenever you have a quiet time to do the exercise will be a good time. It might be in a nice relaxing bubble bath, as you lie in bed just before you go to sleep at night, or even while sitting on the bus on the way home from work. Some people find it easier to do with eyes closed, others find that as soon as they close their eyes they start to go blank. In that case try it with your eyes open. Think of it as like having a positive daydream for two to three minutes.

However, if you can, the absolute best time to do visualisation is after your daily workout and here's why. The mind is most suggestible in two states – one is deep relaxation, which is why hypnotherapy works so well, the other is a state of shock and, intensive exercise shocks your body. If you can take two or three minutes to do your visualisation straight after your exercise session your brain will absorb that new image like a sponge sucks up water – and you'll get faster more effective results.

Step two: take your new blueprint on board

Reprogramming your mind involves giving it a new picture to focus upon, replacing the old image it thought was you. This new image embeds deep into the unconscious mind, snipping away at those long-held beliefs that may be holding you back until eventually they overwrite all the negativity that's driven you to drop diets or regain the weight in the past.

The last section helped you find that image, now we're going to teach you to use it. For two to three minutes every day you're going to do a five-sense visualisation. In these you don't just rely on vision to drive the new image deep into your unconscious, but also integrate the other senses like hearing, touch, taste and smell.

1   Bring up the picture in your head of how you really want to look. If you're finding it hard, take a step back. Imagine looking in the mirror and being reflected back as that image. Still stuck? Take another step back, pretend you're an onlooker viewing yourself looking at that new you in the mirror. Just really see the reflection as you want to. It is not unusual at this point for that gremlin to pop back up saying something negative along the lines of 'Are you kidding yourself?' That's fine, simply let it be and bring your attention back to your picture. The gremlin has no place here and no power to change things.

2   As you see yourself think to yourself 'Wow' – but actually hear yourself speaking the word out loud. Even better, imagine a friend, partner or family member coming in telling you out loud how great you look. Maybe they are asking how you did it. Really hear them speaking in your mind.

3   Focus on the image again – but now also think about how things feel. Start with what you're wearing. Feel how good the clothes feel on your skin. How comfortable they are; how nothing is digging in or tight, maybe the waistbands are even a little loose? Finally think about how your body feels – how flat your tummy is, how firm your arms are, how strong your legs are. Now, think about the emotions you're experiencing. Pride, pleasure, relief, whatever you're experiencing focus on it and how good it feels.

4   Bring your attention back to what you see – now conjure up a scent that surrounds you. Maybe in your image you're walking across a beach showing off your body in a bikini or shorts for the first time. Conjure up the scent of

the sea. Or perhaps you can recall that scent you wore back when you were in your best shape. Feel it filling your nostrils and as the scent intensifies feel your confidence doing the same.

5   Finally, take a drink of water to just stimulate your taste buds. Maybe see it as toasting your success and that new you – sadly you can't do it with real champagne just yet!

Repeat steps one to five two or three times bringing in as many of the senses simultaneously as you can, try and make the whole thing flow like a movie. In Zana's experience, the greater the intensity of everything you see and feel while you do it, the greater the results.

That's all it takes. You may not feel it working, you don't even have to believe it *is* working, but for some people even just one session will be enough to switch the image in your unconscious brain and get it onside as you work towards your goal. For others it will take longer, but so long as every day you keep visualising that same image over and over again it will start to take effect. For best results we recommend practising at least three times a day. Remember, you're trying to chisel a path in your brain that you want it to follow, the more you practise, the clearer the path becomes and eventually all your thoughts will walk along it to your goal.

WHY WE DON'T USE POSITIVE THINKING OR AFFIRMATIONS

Positive thinking sees you repeating statements like 'I am thin, healthy and strong' or 'I can resist temptation'. The theory is if you tell your brain that's the case it will believe you. And it will, if it fits your blueprint and your unconscious believes it too. If it doesn't, whatever words you repeat aren't going to take hold. Not only is this frustrating, the sense of failure and disbelief in your abilities that it creates actually makes us feel worse about ourselves than before, according to researchers from Canada's universities of Waterloo and New Brunswick.[29] It's far more successful to change your unconscious than just trying to convince it with words it doesn't believe.

Step three: silence your inner critic

Ever had that moment when you've been following a diet plan for a while, got on the scales and realised you've lost a pound or a kilo and instead of thinking 'Excellent' had a little voice pipe up and say 'Well that's all right, but considering how much you've got to lose it's not brilliant is it?' That's your inner critic speaking. It's the evil little voice that tells you whatever you're doing isn't good enough. Some psychologists say if you listen closely to that voice you will recognise it. It might be an old teacher, sibling or parent that may have constantly chastised or criticised you as a child. Whoever it is, let's be clear, it's not you. Listening to your inner critic is one of the most soul-destroying things you can do in life. It's exhausting, unfulfilling and it destroys your results.

The joke is there's no way you'd treat someone else in the same situation as badly. Can you imagine if your best friend or teenage son or daughter was trying to lose weight. He or she comes to you and says 'I've lost a pound', at which point instead of congratulating them on their progress, you turn round and say 'Is that all? You've still got ten pounds to go. Maybe you shouldn't have had that extra piece of cheese.

I don't know why you're even bothering.' Yet we say exactly that sort of thing to ourselves over and over again.

We have three ways to quieten the inner voice. First, if it pipes up, talk over it. Find a positive and just keep saying it. Your mind can't think of two things at once and the more you focus it on the positive, the more you drown out the negative. Eventually as the visualisation takes effect the voice will quieten or stop (it's coming from the unconscious after all) but until then, talking over it is the fastest way to stop it speaking.

If this isn't working, the second step is to find something else to do that you really enjoy or completely distracts you. When you are doing something you really enjoy or are fully engaged in, your brain switches into whole brain thinking (a state psychologists call flow), meaning it has no room left over to be thinking anything else! During the Pretox you put together a list of tasks to absorb you. Go back and add to these creating a wealth of interesting or fun things to do when the voice begins. Or if you can find nothing else, play some music you really love, put on your favourite TV show or phone a friend.

Finally, learn to live at least a few moments a day in the present moment. We live our lives planning and assessing, thinking of past events and working out future ones, spending very little, if any, time paying attention to the here and now. Doing so, even for just a few moments really helps you feel calm and happier, making focusing on a positive outcome a lot easier. In addition, however, being able to let go of all those thoughts, even for the briefest period of time, helps reduce stress throughout the day and this stress is often what drives us to make the wrong food choices. So spend a few moments each day simply enjoying the moment, where you are, who you are with and what may be happening in front of and around you. If your mind wanders, as it inevitably will do, simply practise bringing it back to what you see, hear, feel or even smell right, right at that moment.

Not only will this technique help you feel a little more positive and relaxed it can help you let go of the past, even if only for a few minutes. Remember, it is your past experiences and beliefs that actually fuel your inner critic. When you are relaxed and happy, your critic coincidently calms down.

So from today, you're not going to dwell on the past or focus too much on the future, you're going to start enjoying the now. Practise being happy with what you've achieved each day and if you're going to focus on anything in the future focus only on the absolute end result or how what you're doing now is building towards that. After all, if at any given minute of the day what you're doing helps you achieve your goals, the past and future will look after themselves – and before you know it, you will be where you want to be.

Chapter 7

THE MAINTENANCE PLAN

The two weeks of the Pretox, 10-Day Blitz and daily exercise are up, well done! By now you should be noticing a firmer, more toned, slimmer you. Hopefully you're pleased with your results. So now what? There are two options to choose from. You can either decide you'd like to lose some more weight, fat or inches or you can switch your attention to ensuring you keep it off.

IF YOU'D LIKE TO LOSE SOME MORE

If you're enjoying eating the meals on the 10-Day Blitz, stick with it. Zana only recommends 10 days initially as that's a long enough period to really stabilise insulin and achieve great results, but short enough for anyone to do without cheating. You can certainly continue on the plan for longer so long as you continue to follow it perfectly. Remember you can alter the meals by swapping any food in the same group or even make up your own plan using the rules on pages 82–3. You can also eat out so long as you follow our guidelines on pages 84–5.

In terms of continuing to eat such high-fat foods for a little longer, that's not a problem. Yes, trans fats found in processed foods are harmful and you must avoid those, but otherwise, it's the combination of a lot of fat with carbohydrates that's damaging our health and shape. So long as you continue to follow the plan as carefully as before you won't be doing that. You'll be eating your fats from fresh, natural foods and staying away from carbohydrates. Achieve this and you can stay on the plan until you lose all the weight you want. Many of Zana's clients have followed the plan for numerous months and continued to lose weight – one in particular remained on the plan for eight months losing seven stone in the process. The only thing we would suggest if you are going to follow the plan long term is to consider supplementing your diet with a good multivitamin and mineral just to top up your nutrient levels.

However, if you really aren't enjoying the meals or can't see how on earth you can live a normal life while following the plan – or alternatively if at any point when you *are* following it you start to add any carbohydrates – you do need to stop. If you eat carbs on this plan you could gain weight very quickly as your body will come out of ketosis and all those extra calories you're consuming will be stored as fat. You also run the risk of raising cholesterol. This doesn't mean you have to give up the idea of losing more weight though. Simply swap to the Maintenance Plan that follows for a few weeks (some of you may find you continue to lose weight on this too) and whenever you're ready and in the right headspace to fully commit to the 10-Day Blitz again (which will happen) go back on it for another 10 days, or until you shed those last few pounds.

IF YOU'D LIKE TO MAINTAIN YOUR WEIGHT LOSS

This can be the hardest part of any weight-loss plan. There are two reasons it usually doesn't happen. First of all, when people lose weight in many cases over half of what they lose is actually muscle, the very tissue that burns fat and calories helping you keep that lost weight off. Secondly, a 'diet' by its very nature is considered a restricted way of eating for a short space of time, meaning at some point you will have to come off it and eat 'normally'. In doing so, most people simply revert to the old habits that saw them gain extra pounds in the first place. The exercise plan should have eliminated or at least reduced the risk of regain related to muscle loss, so we only have to really tackle the second reason and at this point therefore, Zana suggests you ask yourself a question:

How did you gain the weight you wanted to lose?

The answer may be something short term. For example, the second time Helen went on the plan it was because she had gone to the USA on holiday, ate every burrito she saw and didn't walk a step for a fortnight, gaining 5 lb in the process. Many of Zana's other clients gain due to having a really stressful few months with work and falling into the habit of takeaways and wine. Or, maybe you had friends visiting and have eaten three-course restaurant dinners every night for a week. In other words: if you can clearly pinpoint a short-term overeating blip that has stopped now, but normally you eat well, are at a weight you're happy with and that weight is stable, it's okay to just go back to doing what you did before as chances are the pounds will stay gone, particularly if you keep up the exercise part of the plan and some of the other good habits like watching your carbohydrate intake, limiting alcohol to a few days a week and only eating when you're truly hungry.

If, however, you can't pinpoint a specific reason or event that has caused you to gain the weight – for example, you've always been battling the same stone; your weight has crept up steadily over the last months or years; or you've regained the weight you've lost on every diet you've ever done in the past, then simply going back to eating and exercising the way you used to won't work. If you do this it's very likely that in time all your lost weight will come back.

The purpose of the Maintenance Plan that follows is to help put an end to this. It's a 14-day plan that will teach you to eat in a way that will control your appetite, keep energy levels up and prevent the need for snacking or over-eating. It breaks bad habits and helps you keep the pounds off for good. It consists of medium amounts of natural fats, lots of different proteins and healthy, low-GI carbohydrates. This is the perfect combination to give you a varied, healthy diet that also balances blood sugar and eliminates hunger pangs.

HOW THINGS ARE GOING TO CHANGE

We'll explain this food group by food group in the pages that follow, but as an overview, you're going to be eating lots of healthy proteins, slightly less fat and more leafy green vegetables – but you'll also be adding back in some of the foods that you've eliminated until now, such as fruit, coloured vegetables, dairy and some types of low-GI carbohydrates.

Before you get to the plan though, we'll go through each food group in turn and explain what's changing, why and what foods you should and shouldn't be eating. As with the 10-Day Blitz, some foods may not fall completely into the groups you think they should so do read on.

Fats

A meal with fat is always considerably more satisfying than one without it so you're going to be eating some at virtually every meal, just as you were during the Pretox and 10-Day Blitz. You will notice though that the amount is slightly less than before – about 35–45 g (1.4–1.8 oz) a meal – and it falls even further on days when you're eating starchy carbo-hydrates. On these days you need to be careful of your fat intake. Once you start to eat starchy carbohydrates again calories take on more importance, as any insulin you release will be ready and waiting to shuttle any excess calories into your fat stores. The metabolic advantage you get from eating lots of fat stops when you add carbohydrates to the mix.

Saying that, you should never become afraid of fat. Eaten in the form of natural, fresh, healthy food and in the right proportions it will continue to help keep insulin levels stable, help ensure cravings stay at bay and energy remains high. Quite simply, it's essential to helping you maintain your new weight.

Once you reach Maintenance you can also eat more varie-ties of nuts and seeds. This is because we don't need to keep up such a high ratio of fat vs protein calories to stay in fat-burning mode, so if a nut or seed contains a small percentage of carbohydrates it's not an issue. This means varieties like cashews, peanuts and Brazils are no longer off the menu. You may be surprised to see these listed as fats and not proteins. This is because the majority of their calories come from fat – as much as 66 per cent of the calories in cashew nuts, for example, are from fat.

You might also spot that we've introduced reduced-fat options for some of the dairy foods. This is purely an option for those who find eating the high-fat version of these foods a little hard to handle in terms of digestion or the taste/feel in their mouth. Don't swap to low-fat versions of any other foods though. When companies take fat out of some low-fat foods (yogurts, for example) they often replace it with sugar. The low-fat foods we've added, cream cheese and sour cream, don't have their sugar content significantly altered when fat is removed.

ALLOWED

- Dairy products: butter, clotted cream, crème fraîche, double cream, full-fat cream cheese, full-fat sour cream, mascarpone, reduced-fat cream cheese, reduced-fat sour cream, single cream, whipping cream
- Fruits: avocado
- Nuts: all types are allowed. For example, almonds, Brazil nuts, cashews, coconuts, hazelnuts, macadamia, peanuts, pecans, pine nuts, pistachios, walnuts
- Nut products: CO YO coconut-based yogurt (plain and unsweetened), unsweetened nut butters
- Seeds: any type you like: chia, flax, hemp, linseeds, pumpkin, sesame, sunflower
- Oils: coconut oil, olive oil, any nut oils, ghee

AVOID

- Margarines and low-fat spreads
- Sweetened nut butters
- Low-fat versions of any foods not specifically listed above
- Vegetable oils

Proteins

Depending on the meal you'll be eating 60–180 g (2.4–7.2 oz) of protein-based foods at each meal. This is to help to make your meals more satisfying: combining protein and fat at every meal will supply your body with the fuel it needs for a good four to five hours, helping eliminate cravings for snacks and treats. It will also help you maintain muscle/firm tissue. As mentioned earlier the more muscle you can retain or build in the future the faster your metabolism runs and the easier your weight becomes to control.

You will notice the intake suggested for your evening meal varies from 140–180 g (5.6–7.2 oz). Exactly how much you should consume will depend on your gender, build, how much exercise you do and what form that exercise takes. Anyone training with reasonable intensity for more than 45 minutes a day – and looking to maintain their muscle mass – needs more protein. Men, particularly those looking to build size with weight training, should also err towards the higher intake starting at 180 g (7.2 oz) each evening listening to your body to determine if you need less or a little more. On the other hand, if you're not a heavy exerciser, dipping down lower than we suggest to 120 g (4.8 oz) may be enough long term. Your body will tell you what it needs. If you feel too full on large portions cut back. However, if you find you are genuinely hungry or craving sugar in the middle of the afternoon or evening, chances are you didn't eat enough protein earlier, so increase your protein intake 20 g (0.8 oz) at the relevant meal and ensure you are taking in the right amount of fats.

Because we don't have to reach the high fat to protein calorie ratio as we did before you no longer have to add fat to the lower-fat proteins. This relaxing of the rules also allows us to add moderate amounts of other dairy products such as Greek yogurt or full-fat natural yogurt as well as small amounts of full-fat milk all of which had too little fat and too much lactose (natural milk sugar) to be included before now. Steer clear of other yogurts though, a lot of them contain added sugars on top of their natural ones – in fact, an average low-fat fruit yogurt can contain the equivalent of as many as five teaspoons of sugar. One thing you really want to avoid from now on is any kind of added sugar.

ALLOWED

- Eggs: organic/free-range duck, hen, quail
- Pork: including bacon (no added sugar and nitrate free), chorizo (no added sugar and nitrate free), gammon, pancetta, Parma ham, pork belly, pork chops, pork fillet, ribs (no sauce), tenderloin
- Beef: burgers if 100 per cent beef, mince, roasting, ribs (no sauce), steak – particularly rib-eye or sirloin, veal
- Lamb: all cuts including breast, chops, leg, mince, neck, rack, rump, shanks, shoulder
- Poultry: any organic or free-range chicken, breast, drumsticks, livers, thighs or wings. Duck, turkey, turkey mince, goose
- Game: venison, rabbit
- Dairy: casein-protein powder, full-fat Greek yogurt, reduced-fat Greek yogurt, milk – in small amounts, preferably full fat; cheeses such as Brie, Camembert, cottage cheese, Gorgonzola, Emmental, Gruyère, halloumi, Roquefort, Stilton or blue cheese
- Fish: all white fish like cod, haddock, sole, pollock; tuna canned in brine or spring water; oily fish such as anchovies, eel, fresh salmon, fresh tuna, herring, kippers, mackerel, pilchards, sardines, smoked salmon, trout, tuna canned in oil, whitebait
- Shellfish: crab, mussels and prawns
- Offal: heart, kidneys, liver
- Vegetable proteins: tofu, TVP, Quorn

Starchy carbohydrates

They are back – very occasionally though. At most you should be eating starchy carbohydrates at two meals a week, in a portion size of 50–75 g (2–3 oz) – and ideally they are best with your evening meal. By focusing your carbohydrate intake around evening meals, when you do eat them you at least control the amount of 'damage' the increased insulin can do to your waistline. If you miss toast with your break-fast eggs though, a slice of a low-GI bread like rye or teff bread in the morning now and again is okay too. Just don't fall back into the trap of eating too many starchy carbohydrates or any amount of sugary ones in the morning. It is important to get your first meal of the day right. If you start your day with an insulin surge it is very difficult to stabilise it again over the course of the day. This can lead to an increased risk of fat storage – and you could find yourself craving sugars.

Every carbohydrate raises blood sugar so for health and weight you should be aiming to choose those that raise it least. That means you will be trying to mostly eat carbohydrates with a low or medium rating on the glycaemic index. How high a carbohydrate rates on the GI scale can depend on a few things including:

- How much fibre it contains. Fibre makes food harder to digest so it releases sugars more slowly. Granary versions of bread, for example, have a lower GI than white bread does.
- Is it cooked or raw? The sugars in raw food are harder to access than those in cooked food. This is why pasta cooked al dente has a lower GI than that cooked with less bite.
- Has it been processed to make it easier to digest? Foods where the starch is partly broken down can be more quickly turned into sugar by the body and so have a higher GI. Instant porridges to which you can just add water, for example, have a higher GI than steel-cut porridge oats, which have to be cooked for a long period before they soften.

One thing that might surprise you is to see beans and pulses in the list below – especially if you are vegetarian and are used to using these as a source of protein in your diet. It's true they are good sources of protein, but most of the calories they contain come from carbohydrates, 70 per cent of the calories in lentils and 73 per cent of those in kidney beans, for example. As such we class them as carbohydrates.

ALLOWED

- Breads: granary bread, rye bread, sourdough, teff bread
- Crackers: oat cakes, rye crackers
- Pasta and noodles: all types of wholewheat pasta – but ideally choose thicker shapes – and cook it al dente, glass noodles, kelp noodles, konjac noodles, soba noodles, udon noodles

- Cereals: All Bran, steel-cut oats, unsweetened muesli
- Grains: barley, buckwheat, bulgar wheat, couscous, freekah, quinoa, teff
- Potatoes and tubers (cooked whole): new potatoes, sweet potatoes, yams
- Rice: basmati rice, brown rice, red rice, wild rice
- Beans and pulses: black beans, butter beans, cannellini beans, chickpeas, kidney beans, lentils, pinto beans, soy beans

AVOID

- Breads: brown breads or white breads of any kind including baguettes, bagels, ciabatta and tortilla wraps
- Crackers: matzo, rice cakes
- Pasta and noodles: gluten-free pasta, white or over-cooked pasta of any kind, rice noodles
- Cereals: any processed cereals or kinds of flake, anything with honey or sugar, instant porridge, puffed cereals
- Grains: amaranth, millet
- Potatoes and tubers: any white potato other than new potatoes, mashed sweet potatoes
- Rice: jasmine rice, quick-cook rice, sticky rice, white rice

Vegetables

You're going to be eating up to five portions a day of around 50–60 g each (2–2.4 oz) during Maintenance. As before though we're going to be asking you to eat mostly green or white vegetables to have the lowest impact on your insulin levels.

The good news is we've added a few more to them, including the less starchy root vegetables like radishes and mooli.

This doesn't mean the colours are neglected though – once or twice a week swap one of your green/white vegetables for any of the choices on our second list. Once the 14-days are up if you want to eat a portion of brighter vegetables daily that's no problem, but keep them raw or lightly cooked where appropriate as this slows their digestion and effect on insulin slightly. Keep the majority of your vegetables those green and white staples, however. It's also okay to increase portion sizes of these after Maintenance – 80 g (3.2 oz) is recommended by the World Health Organization as the portion size you should aim for.

VEGETABLE JUICES

Any juicing results in the consumption of a far greater quantity of the food, and you also lose all the fibre that slows the speed with which it turns into sugar. This in turn leads to a rapid rise in blood sugar and insulin. That said, green vegetable juices, in particular those that include an avocado, will have a much lower GI than fruit juices. Our recommendation is to leave vegetable juices out for this part of the plan, however, if you do wish to reintroduce in the future, keep them to no more than two to three times a week.

ALLOWED DAILY

Alfalfa sprouts, all lettuce, artichokes, asparagus, aubergine, bamboo shoots, beansprouts, bok choy, broccoli, broccolini, broad beans, Brussels sprouts, cauliflower, cavolo nero, celery, chicory, chilli peppers, courgette, cucumber, edamame, fennel, green beans, green pepper, jalapenos, kale, leeks, marrow, mooli, mushrooms, okra, peas, radish, rocket, runner beans, samphire, savoy cabbage, seaweed, spinach, spring greens, spring onions, Swiss chard, watercress, white cabbage

ALLOWED ONE TO TWO TIMES A WEEK

Beetroot, butternut squash, carrots, celeriac, onions, parsnips, pumpkin, radicchio, red cabbage, red peppers, shallots, turnip, yellow peppers

Fruits

If you've been missing biting into a crisp juicy apple or the sweet taste of a punnet of blueberries you'll be glad to hear that fruit also makes a comeback – you can have up to one portion a day, particularly of the slightly more sour fruits like those in the citrus family and berries. Acidity also lowers the GI rating of a food and so the more sour a fruit tastes, the lower its impact on your blood sugar.

When it comes to other fruit, the less sweet the better – choose fruits local to the UK like apples (particularly Cox and Braeburn varieties) and eat sweeter fruit like pears, peaches, apricots and plums before they become soft and overripe. If you want more tropical fruits, keep them as a treat and ideally eat them as part of a fruit salad sprinkled with a little lemon juice or topped with something containing a little fat like crème fraîche, both of which lower the GI of a meal.

Avoid fruit-based juices or smoothies though. The sheer amount of fruit you need to create even a small glass of juice is far more than you would comfortably eat normally. To make one 225 ml (9 fl oz) glass of orange juice, for example, actually takes three medium oranges. When you juice a fruit you also lose all the fibre that slows the speed with which it turns into sugar. Fruit juices therefore lead to a rapid rise in blood sugar and insulin.

ALLOWED REGULARLY

Apples, blackberries, blackcurrants, blueberries, cherries, grapefruit, lemon, lime, olives, oranges, raspberries. Slightly less ripe apricots, plums, kiwi, peaches and pears

ALLOWED OCCASIONALLY

Cantaloupe, grapes, mango, papaya, pineapple, tomato, watermelon. Ripe versions of apricots, peaches, pears, plums, etc.

AVOID

Any fruit canned in syrup. Dried fruit like dates, figs, raisins or sultanas, fruit-based juices and smoothies

Herbs, spices, dressings and condiments

All fresh herbs and spices are allowed as they were on the Pretox and 10-Day Blitz plan, but what changes now is that you can introduce a few more ready-made condiments and other flavourings to the mix. While you're still trying to stay away from anything with high levels of added sugar (like ketchup), because you're no longer in ketosis the small levels of carbohydrates added to some other flavourings won't have as negative an impact on your waistline as they might on the 10-Day Blitz, this means you can introduce some things you have been avoiding like stocks, ready-made pesto or mayonnaise. Formulations do vary wildly though so before you pour, spritz or splash anything into a dish or on to your salad, the key is to read the label. Anything with less than 2 g (0.7 oz) of sugar per 100 g (4 oz) serving is okay, more than that still steer clear.

ALLOWED

Bay leaves, capers, cayenne pepper, cider vinegar, chilli flakes, chilli powder, coriander, chives, cinnamon, cumin, Dijon mustard or any mustard with no added sugar, dill, fresh chillies, fresh horseradish, fresh wasabi, garlic, ginger, lemon juice, lime juice, malt vinegar, mayonnaise, mint, mustard powder, nutmeg, oregano, Oxo cubes, paprika, parsley, pepper, ready-made pesto, red wine vinegar, rosemary, salt, stock cubes, Tabasco, tapenade, thyme, turmeric, vinegar, white vinegar

AVOID

Agave, balsamic vinegar, BBQ sauce, English mustard or any other form with added sugar, fish sauce, honey, ketchup, mirin, miso, salad cream, soy sauce, sweet chilli sauce, tamari, teriyaki, tomato purée. Any prepared sauce, dressing or rub that has more than 2 g (0.08 oz) of sugar per 100 g (4 oz)

Drinks

Because most drinks are very sugary, not much is going to change between the Pretox, the 10-Day Blitz and here, although you might find you don't get as thirsty so don't need to drink as often because you're eating more fruit and vegetables.

You're probably wondering about diet drinks. Ideally you want to avoid processed foods so don't bring them back as a daily habit. It is possible to create some tasty drinks without resorting to processed concoctions. We've included some ideas on pages 242–3.

You can, however, add a small amount of milk to your tea and coffee now, replacing the cream or butter. Ideally choose full-fat or semi-skimmed milks and avoid skimmed varieties, as fat will slow how fast lactose, the sugar in milk, enters your bloodstream. If you like the cream or butter though, keep it up but for no more than one cup a day. Remember you will no longer have the metabolic advantage to rely on so calories do count a little more and if you consume a few hundred extra in the form of creamy coffee you could start to gain weight.

For the 14 days of Maintenance we will still ask you to avoid alcohol but that doesn't mean this is for life.

ALLOWED

Black coffee/tea, herbal teas, green tea, hot water with coconut oil, sparkling water, still water, tea/coffee with butter, tea/coffee with coconut oil, tea/coffee with double cream, unsweetened soy or almond milk

AVOID

Alcohol, bottled water with sugars, coconut milk, coconut water, flavoured milk drinks, fizzy drinks (including diet versions), juices including vegetable juices, milky coffees, oat milk, probiotic drinks, rice milk, smoothies, sweetened nut milks, sweetened soy milk, squashes and cordials

Snacks

Sorry to build your hopes up there – there is ideally no snacking on this plan at all, not even on things like fruit.

The idea that we need to snack is directly related to our low-fat, high-sugar, highly refined carb diets. When you eat a diet packed full of these foods your blood-sugar levels yo-yo so frequently that your body is constantly crying out for more food to provide it with energy. Eat proper meals two or three times a day, always including some protein and some fat, and you won't actually need to snack. If do you feel genuinely hungry or suffer cravings while on this plan, check your fat intake and increase the amount of protein you're consuming rather than reaching for extra snacks/meals to fill the gap and this will normally resolve the issue. If, however, you *really* still feel the need to eat between meals then have something that contains a little protein and fat – e.g. a slice of cheese with four or five walnuts. Treat this as a small meal and don't start to graze all day.

Of course, psychological cravings for food are very different from genuine hunger. If you're snacking because you're bored, tired, sad, stressed or any other emotional reason it won't matter how much fat and protein you eat you'll still need to fill that hole. Knowing that you're eating emotionally is the first stage in fighting this and to help identify if you are, it's good to know the differences between physical and emotional hunger.

Physical hunger comes on slowly; emotional hunger comes on very quickly.

Physical hunger can be satisfied with any food; emotional hunger is often linked to a specific food or type of food.

Physical hunger has physical symptoms: a growling tummy, feeling light-headed, low energy; emotional hunger doesn't.

If you do eat emotionally it's important to address this. You need to start associating food with health, vitality and fuelling your body, rather than as a way to tackle your emotions. Find new ways to deal with emotional stress or boredom. Adding yoga classes or mindfulness techniques to your weekly regime can also help you develop a calmer more controlled emotional state rather than one that reacts unfavourably to things going on around you.

Practising the techniques in Chapter 6 will also help you gain more control over emotional eating. Remember, if you reprogramme your unconscious so it thinks you should be the new slim shape it sees in the mirror it'll make it more likely that your new automatic reaction to stress or upset is not to raid the fridge but to go for a walk or call a friend.

WHAT ABOUT EXERCISE?

Keep it up. The more muscle you can create in the future the more effective your metabolism will become long term, really helping you keep that weight off forever. You don't have to work out daily though. If you're doing the High Intensity Gym Workout, cut back to three or a maximum of five times a week; if you're doing the High Intensity Home Workout cut back to four to five days a week. Still work with the same speed and intensity, moving quickly between the exercises and still lifting the heaviest weights you can with good form. That's the key to success with the programme.

At this point if you want to start doing more traditional cardiovascular workouts again you can. They aren't necessary to maintain your results but they will aid circulation and overall health. Try not to do more than 40 minutes in any one session, however. Remember, this is the point at which exercise starts to break down muscle faster than you can replace it and therefore long training sessions can actually lower your metabolism. It will also help to add some sessions of high-intensity interval training (HIIT) rather than focusing solely on steady state cardio. HIIT is best done under the supervision of an instructor and sees you combining short bursts of maximum intensity with periods of recovery – for example, 30 seconds of sprinting or rapid cycling and 30–60 seconds of slower jogging or steady pedalling. This type of training can trigger a greater fat loss than steady training of lesser intensity and also creates a high release of human growth hormone helping preserve muscle.

Those of you who do enjoy running or cycling long distance, that's okay but you may want to alter your training slightly from that which you're used to. Keep up the High Intensity Gym Workout twice a week, or do the High Intensity Home Workout two to three times a week. Add to this one to two sessions a week of running or cycling that are under 40 minutes and then a final longer session once a week. In addition keep to the higher intakes of protein suggested in the eating plan to help ensure muscle recovery rather than breakdown – and definitely look into supplements to help protect the joints and ensure muscle recovery, like extra omega-3 oils which help reduce inflammation; glucosamine sulphate which helps with the repair of tissue damage; casein protein, which helps ensure sufficient protein to nourish and repair the muscle, and finally magnesium, which helps keep muscles relaxed reducing post-training soreness and cramping.

If you've developed a liking for weights and a stronger-looking body that's great too. If you're now interested in creating serious bulk you might be wondering how the plan is going to affect your ability to do so. Can you really do it with such a short workout? The answer is yes – the principles are the same. For best results you will certainly need to use the High Intensity Gym Workout but focus only on one body part (i.e. chest or back, shoulders or arms, or legs) per day. Do four exercises on that part using exactly the same intensity and repetition protocol but repeat it for four to five sets, not just three. That will get you results, but please remember that the majority of change in terms of muscle size will come from nutrition rather than training. To increase bulk you may need to dramatically increase your protein intake so that you are consuming a minimum of 400 g (16 oz) of protein foods with your evening meal. In addition, insulin in this case is actually very helpful for driving protein into the muscle so increase your carbohydrate intake to once every two or three days.

THE MAINTENANCE DIET PLAN

The plan that follows gives you suggestions of meals for the next 14 days. If you want to keep it up after that then simply repeat it, or, even better start mixing and matching your own meals using the lists of foods in the pages before this as that will help you develop your own good habits for life. Also, don't forget you can also swap any ingredients from the same food groups. We have tried to appeal to everyone on this plan and so use lots of different foods, particularly when it comes to accompaniments like vegetables, but following it exactly, especially if you're catering for just one person, could leave you with a lot of food waste. Try and account for the smaller portions when you are shopping and buy only what you think you need, but also feel free to swap any suggested vegetable (or other food) for another in the same food group to reduce waste. As with the plans that have gone before it, also don't feel you have to eat all the meals – or our recommended portion sizes – if you're not hungry.

Can I stay on the plan for longer?

Absolutely, the idea is that this is how you eat for life so you can repeat it as many times as you like until you feel confident enough to start making up your own meals.

MAINTENANCE: THE PLAN

Day 1

BREAKFAST

Creamy mushrooms made from mixing 50–60 g (2–2.4 oz) sliced mushrooms with 45 g (1.8 oz) melted full-fat cream cheese. Serve with 60 g (2.4 oz) grilled bacon or sliced chorizo

Or

150 g (5 oz) Greek yogurt served with 30 g (1.2 oz) blueberries or raspberries and 45 g (1.8 oz) any nut you like

LUNCH

90 g (3.6 oz) Parma ham spread with 45 g (1.8 oz) full-fat cream cheese. Wrap round 50–60 g (2–2.4 oz) lightly steamed asparagus spears and serve with 50–60 g (2–2.4 oz) rocket

Or

Steak and feta salad (see recipe on page 228)

EVENING MEAL

120–140 g (4.3–5 oz) grilled sole or haddock topped with 50–60 g (2–2.2 oz) sliced leeks cooked in 15 g (0.6 oz) butter with garlic. Serve with 50–75 g (2–3 oz) roasted sweet potato and 50–60 g (2–2.4 oz) broccoli

Or

50–75 g (2–3 oz) pasta spirals, cooked al dente, tossed with 50–60 g (2–2.4 oz) courgette and 50–60 g (2–2.2 oz) broccoli and 15 g (0.6 oz) of warmed full- or low-fat cream cheese. Top with a 120–140 g (4.3–5 oz) mix of prawns and crabmeat

Day 2

BREAKFAST

Two poached eggs served with 50–60 g (2–2.4 oz) grilled mushrooms pan-fried in 25 g (1 oz) butter. Add 20 g (0.8 oz) walnuts or pumpkin seeds

Or

One serving of chia porridge (see recipe on page 225) topped with 20 g (0.8 oz) CO YO yogurt or crème fraîche

LUNCH

90 g (3.6 oz) buffalo mozzarella served with half an avocado on a bed of 50–60 g (2–2.4 oz) chopped lettuce and half a medium green pepper, sliced

Or

Omelette made from 2 eggs, 30 g (1.2 oz) diced cooked chicken or sliced grilled bacon and 45 g (1.8 oz) of Boursin cheese. Serve with 50–60 g (2–2.4 oz) courgettes

EVENING MEAL

140–180 g (5–6.4 oz) grilled salmon fillet served with 100–120 g (3.5–4 oz) cauliflower mashed with 35 g (1.4 oz) cream cheese or crème fraîche

Or

1–2 lamb or beef burgers (see recipe on page 102) topped with 50–60 g (2–2.4 oz) diced onion fried in 10 g (0.4 oz) butter. Serve with salad of 50–60 g (2–2.4 oz) rocket and 50g (2 oz) avocado

BREAKFAST

2 eggs scrambled with 25 g (1 oz) of butter and 20 g (0.8 oz) cream cheese

Or

60 g (2.2 oz) Emmental or Gruyère cheese. One apple. Serve with a side of 45 g (1.8 oz) CO YO yogurt or 45 g (1.8 oz) any nut or seed

LUNCH

Creamy chicken and celery soup (see recipe on page 229). Serve with 30 g (1.2 oz) walnuts

Or

One green pepper halved and deseeded filled with 90 g (3.6 oz) smoked or fresh salmon mixed with 45 g (1.8 oz) full-fat cream cheese or crème fraîche. Serve with 2–3 chopped green olives

EVENING MEAL

140–180 g (5–6.4 oz) roast lamb, served with 50–60 g (2–2.4 oz) Brussels sprouts and 50–60 g (2–2.4 oz) peas mashed with 35 g (1.4 oz) crème fraîche or cream cheese with a little mint

Or

140–180 g (5–6.4 oz) mix of prawns and scallops sautéed with garlic in 20 g (0.8 oz) butter. Serve with 50–60 g (2–2.4 oz) spinach and a small green salad with 15 g (0.6 oz) toasted pine nuts and some parmesan shavings

Day 4

BREAKFAST

60 g (2.4 oz) smoked salmon with 45 g (1.8 oz) full-fat cream cheese and 50–60 g (2–2.2 oz) spinach

Or

60 g (2.4 oz) cottage cheese served alongside 45 g (1.8 oz) mixed nuts including walnuts, pine nuts, almonds and cashews

LUNCH

Large green salad 100–120 g (4- 4.8 oz) dressed with one tablespoon of olive oil and lemon juice. Serve with 90 g (3.6 oz) fresh sardines (or other oily fish) and 30 g (1.2 oz) any nut or seed

Or

90 g (3.6 oz) grilled steak or sliced roast beef (ready cooked from the supermarket but check the sugar) on a bed of 50–60 g (2–2.4 oz) rocket and 50–60 g (2–2.4 oz) grilled red peppers. Top with 50–60 g (2–2.4 oz) mushrooms cooked with garlic and 15 g (0.6 oz) butter. Add 40 g (1.6 oz) cream cheese or half an avocado

EVENING MEAL

115–155 g (4.1–5.5 oz) of any white fish, pan-fried. Serve with 50–60 g (2–2.4 oz) of leeks stir-fried with 25 g (1 oz) chopped bacon or pancetta and top with 35 g (1.4 oz) melted cream cheese sauce or pine nuts

Or

Peppered lamb steaks with creamy mushroom sauce (see recipe on page 230) served with 50–60 g (2–2.4 oz) courgetti (see recipe on page 240)

BREAKFAST

Baked eggs (see recipe on page 227

Or

One serving of chia porridge (see recipe on page 225) served with 20 g (0.8 oz) crème fraîche or double cream

LUNCH

Feta and avocado dip (see recipe on page 231) served with 50 g (2 oz) king prawns (grilled or pre-cooked) and a side salad of 50–60 g (2–2.4 oz) cucumber and mint

Or

Two slices 50–60 g (2–2.4 oz) each of aubergine, grilled topped with 60 g (2.4 oz) fresh or canned tuna in oil and one boiled egg mixed with one tablespoon mayonnaise. Serve with 30 g (1.2 oz) any nut or seed

EVENING MEAL

140–180 g (5–6.4 oz) grilled sole or haddock served on a bed of 100–120 g (4–4.8 oz) sliced mushrooms fried with 10 g (0.4 oz) butter and garlic. Sprinkle with 25 g (1 oz) pine nuts and serve with 50–60 g (2–2.2 oz) rocket drizzled with a little olive oil and lemon juice

Or

140–180 g (5–6.4 oz) roast lamb or pork served with 100–120 g (4–4.8 oz) kale or savoy cabbage sautéed in 35 g (1.4 oz) coconut oil with chilli

BREAKFAST

60 g (2.4 oz) Emmental cheese with 45 g (1.8 oz) almonds, walnuts or cashews and one sliced apple

Or

2 poached eggs served on one slice of toasted rye or pumpernickel bread with half an avocado

LUNCH

90 g (3.6 oz) fresh salmon (ready cooked from the supermarket is okay) served on 50–60 g (2–2.4 oz) broccoli florets steamed and tossed in one tablespoon of Zana's dressing (see recipe on page 106) or with 45 g (1.8 oz) mixed seeds

Or

90 g (3.6 oz) grilled lamb or sliced roast beef skewered with 50–60 g (2–2.4 oz) courgettes or cucumber and mushrooms. Serve with a dip of 45 g (1.8 oz) sour cream mixed with 1–2 teaspoons chopped fresh dill

EVENING MEAL

120–140 g (4.8–5.6 oz) grilled chicken served with 50–75 g (2–3 oz) new potatoes mixed with one tablespoon mayonnaise and a little spring onion. Serve with 50–60 g (2–2.4 oz) buttered green beans

Or

Seafood basmati (see recipe on page 234)

BREAKFAST

1 egg poached, serve with 30 g (1.2 oz) pan-fried sliced chorizo on a bed of half an avocado mashed

Or

150 g (5 oz) Greek yogurt mixed with 25 g (1 oz) walnuts and 20 g (0.8 oz) cashew nuts

LUNCH

90 g (3.6 oz) grilled halloumi cheese on a salad of 50–60 g (2–2.4 oz) spinach, rocket or lettuce, 50–60 g (2–2.2 oz) celery or cucumber and 45 g (1.8 oz) of any nut or seed

Or

90 g (3.6 oz) sliced turkey breast with 40 g (1.6 oz) avocado and 25 g (1 oz) pine nuts served on a bed of 100–120 g (4–4.8 oz) green salad

EVENING MEAL

Creamy ratatouille with grilled salmon (see recipe on page 232)

Or

140–180 g (5–6.4 oz) steak, cut into strips and stir-fried in 10 g (0.4 oz coconut oil) with 50–60 g (2–2.4 oz) sliced green or red pepper, ginger and garlic. Serve on a bed of 100–120 g (4–4.8 oz) kale or cabbage with 25 g (1 oz) cashew nuts

Day 8

BREAKFAST

One serving of chia porridge (see recipe on page 225) with 20g (0.8 oz) crème fraîche or CO YO yogurt

Or

Omelette made from two eggs and 45 g (1.8 oz) melted full-fat cream cheese. Add 50–60 g (2–2.4 oz) sliced mushrooms, courgettes or spinach

LUNCH

100–120 g (4–4.2 oz) chopped romaine lettuce drizzled with Zana's salad dressing (see recipe page 106) or 1 tablespoon mayonnaise. Top with 90 g (3.6 oz) grilled (or pre-cooked) prawns or chicken pieces and 20 g (0.8 oz) pine nuts and sesame seeds

Or

90 g (3.6 oz) smoked salmon served with 50–60 g (2–2.4 oz) watercress and 50–60 g (2–2.4 oz) cucumber ribbons and 1 tablespoon sour cream mixed with 25 g (1 oz) walnuts or pumpkin seeds

EVENING MEAL

140–180 g (5–6.4 oz) roasted pork served with 50–60 g (2–2.4 oz) kale or cabbage sautéed in 10 g (0.8 oz) butter or coconut oil and a side of cauliflower rice (see recipe on page 239). Add 25 g (1 oz) pine nuts to the rice

Or

140–180 g (5–6.4 oz) tuna, grilled. Serve on a bed of a 100–120 g (4–4.8 oz) mix of stir-fried bok choy, mushrooms and beansprouts. Add 35 g (1.4 oz) cashew nuts

Day 9

BREAKFAST

One apple, sliced. Spoon out 45 g (1.8 oz) unsweetened or homemade peanut butter (see recipes on page 238) and use as a dip for the apple. Serve with 60 g (2.4 oz) Emmental cheese

Or

60 g (2.4 oz) grilled streaky bacon with 50–60 g (2–2.2 oz) grilled mushrooms, add half an avocado

LUNCH

Two or three eggs boiled then mashed with one tablespoon of mayonnaise and 25 g (1 oz) pine nuts. Serve on a bed of 50–60 g (2–2.4 oz) watercress with 50–60 g (2–2.4 oz) cucumber

Or

90 g (3.6 oz) Parma ham or smoked salmon slices. Roll around 50–60 g (2–2.4 oz) lightly steamed asparagus spears. Serve with 50–60 g (2–2.4 oz) rocket

EVENING MEAL

Cauliflower bake (see recipe on page 233) served with 120–160 g (4.2–5.7 oz) chicken and half a small avocado

Or

140–180 g (5–6.4 oz) white fish like sole, cod or pollock pan-fried with red chilli and ginger in one tablespoon olive or coconut oil. Serve with 50–60 g (2–2.4 oz) C-oodles (see recipe on page 240) mixed with 20 g (0.8 oz) pine nuts

BREAKFAST

1 poached egg, 30 g (1.2 oz) Parma ham and 50–60 g (2–2.4 oz) of spinach cooked with 45 g (1.8 oz) Boursin cheese

Or

Raspberry and walnut parfait (see recipe on page 226)

LUNCH

90 g (3.6 oz) of chicken served with a coleslaw made from 100–120 g (4–4.8 oz) mix of shredded cabbage, celery and fennel and one tablespoon of mayonnaise. Add 20 g (0.8 oz) of any nut or seed

Or

90 g (3.6 oz) raw or pan-fried tuna or salmon canned in oil served on a bed of sliced mushrooms and half an avocado with 50–60 g (2–2.4 oz) lettuce

EVENING MEAL

140–180 g (5–6.4 oz) sole, cod or haddock grilled. Serve with 50–60 g (2–2.2 oz) spinach and one large grilled Portobello mushroom topped with 25 g (1 oz) melted full-fat cream cheese and 10 g (0.4 oz) of crushed nuts

Or

Spicy lamb meatballs (see recipe on page 99 but serve without the tzatziki) served with courgetti (see recipe on page 240) and half an avocado

Day 11

BREAKFAST

2 eggs poached, serve with half a sliced avocado and 50–60 g (2–2.4 oz) spinach

Or

150 g (7 oz) Greek yogurt with 40 g (1.6 oz) mixed berries

LUNCH

Fill 3 large lettuce leaves with a mix of 90 g (3.6 oz) sardines or mackerel and 25 g (1 oz) chopped onion mixed with 1 tablespoon mayonnaise. Serve with 50–60 g (2–2.4 oz) cucumber and 30 g (1.2 oz) of any nut or seed

Or

90 g (3.6 oz) king prawns (grilled or pre-cooked), skewered into kebabs with half an avocado. Serve on a bed of 100–120 g (4–4.8 oz) rocket and cucumber

EVENING MEAL

Chicken and black beans (see recipe on page 235). Serve with 50–60 g (2–2.4 oz) green beans

Or

120–140 g (4.3–5 oz) grilled fresh tuna. Serve with one sliced sweet potato roasted in olive oil or coconut oil and 50–60 g (2–2.4 oz) garden peas cooked in 10 g (0.4 oz) butter. Add 2–3 mint leaves to garnish

BREAKFAST

1 egg scrambled, add 30 g (1.2 oz) sliced, pan-fried chorizo and serve with 45 g (1.6 oz) pumpkin seeds

Or

30 g (1.2 oz) crème fraîche or plain, unsweetened CO YO yogurt. Serve with 60 g (2.4 oz) cottage or feta cheese, 1 apple topped with 15 g (0.6 oz) peanut butter

LUNCH

One serving of cooled cauliflower rice (see recipe on page 239) with 25 g (1 oz) pine nuts. Add 90 g (3.6 oz) flaked cooked salmon and drizzle with olive oil or lemon juice. Serve with 50–60 g (2–2.4 oz) cucumber batons dipped into 20 g (0.8 oz) cream cheese

Or

90 g (3.6 oz) buffalo mozzarella diced and mixed with 50–60 g (2–2.4 oz) chopped green olives. Serve on a bed of 50–60 g (2–2.4 oz) baby spinach and half an avocado. Add a dressing of olive oil and cider vinegar if desired

EVENING MEAL

Cod wrapped in Parma ham (see recipe on page 236) served with 50–60 g (2–2.4 oz) spinach mixed with 30 g (1.2 oz) crème fraîche or cream cheese. 50–60 g (2–2.4 oz) green beans

Or

140–180 g (5–6.4 oz) pork stir-fried in 10 g (0.8 oz) coconut oil with 100–120 g (4–4.2 oz) mix of beansprouts, green pepper and bok choy. Add chilli and ginger and 25 g (1 oz) cashew nuts

Day 13

BREAKFAST

30 g (1.2 oz) flaked cooked herring, smoked haddock or salmon with 1 egg scrambled with 25 g (1 oz) butter and 20 g (0.8 oz) cream cheese

Or

60 g (2.4 oz) back or streaky bacon, grilled with 50–60 g (2–2.4 oz) mushrooms and 45 g (1.8 oz) of any nut or seed

LUNCH

Turkey club: alternate slices of 45 g (1.8 oz) sliced turkey breast with 45 g (1.8 oz) Cheddar or Emmental cheese. Serve on a bed of lettuce with half an avocado

Or

90 g (3.6 oz) tinned salmon mixed with one tablespoon mayonnaise served in 2–3 large lettuce leaves and 30 g (1.2 oz) pumpkin seeds or walnuts

EVENING MEAL

140–180 g (5–6.4 oz) white fish, pan-fried served with carrot chips (see recipe on page 241) and 50–60 g (2–2.4 oz) peas and a sauce of 25 g (1 oz) melted cream cheese

Or

140–180 g (5–6.4 oz) pork chop, grilled. Serve on a bed of 50–60 g (2–2.4 oz) spinach leaves with half a diced avocado. Add 50–60 g (2–2.4 oz) diced red and yellow pepper mixed with some chopped fresh coriander and lime juice

BREAKFAST

150 g (5 oz) Greek yogurt mixed with 45 g (1.8 oz) of unsweetened, or homemade, nut butter. 30–40 g (1.2–1.6 oz) berries

Or

1 egg and yolk fried in one tablespoon olive oil, 30 g (1.2 oz) grilled bacon and 60 g (2.4 oz) avocado

LUNCH

90 g (3.6 oz) fresh mackerel (grilled or try a ready-cooked fillet from the supermarket) served on a bed of watercress with a tablespoonful of horseradish sauce (see recipe on page 109). Add 30 g (1.2 oz) walnuts or half a small avocado

Or

Omelette or frittata made from 2 eggs and 30 g (1.2 oz) grated Cheddar cheese. Serve with 50–60 g (2–2.4 oz) rocket and 45 g (1.8 oz) of any nut or seed

EVENING MEAL

140–180 g (5–6.4 oz) rib-eye steak served with 50–60 g (2–2.4 oz) broccoli tossed with 25 g (1 oz) pine nuts and 50–60 g (2–2.4 oz) mushrooms fried in 10 g (0.8 oz) butter or olive oil

Or

Cauliflower-topped shepherd's pie (see recipe on page 237) served with buttered green beans

HOW TO PLAN YOUR OWN MEALS

As with the 10-Day Blitz, the meals on the Maintenance Plan are great ideas to get you started but it's very easy to create meals of your own. Here are the rules to follow.

If you're having three meals a day

BREAKFAST

Have up to 60 g (2.4 oz) of any fish, meat or cheese in the protein list or two organic or free-range eggs. If you like to start your day with Greek yogurt, have 150 g (5 oz). Serve this with 45 g (1.8 oz) of any foods from the fats list – or, if choosing avocado have half of a Hass-sized fruit. If you want to you can also add 30–40 g (1.2–1.6 oz) fruit or 50–60 g (2–2.4 oz) vegetables.

LUNCH

Serve 90 g (3.6 oz) of any food on the protein list. Add 45 g (1.8 oz) of any foods from the fats list or, if choosing avocado have half of a Hass-sized fruit. Serve up to two 50–60 g (2–2.2 oz) portions of vegetables – particularly those from the allowed list.

EVENING MEAL

If it's a normal day, serve 140–180 g (5–6.4 oz) of any protein on the list with 35 g (1.4 oz) of any fat from the list or, if choosing avocado have half of a Hass-sized fruit and two 50–60 g (2–2.2 oz) portions of vegetables.

If it's a carbohydrate day, reduce protein to 120–140 g (4.3–5 oz). Add a 50–75 g (2–3 oz) serving of any food from the carbohydrate list, serve with 15 g (0.6 oz) of any food from the fats list, or 30 g (1.2 oz) avocado and one or two 50–60g (2–2.2 oz) servings of vegetables.

It's also okay to adapt parts of meals in the plan, if for example, you need to use up some vegetables or have some extra chicken leftover. You can swap any item in the plan for any other item from the same food group.

If you decide you work better on two meals a day

Many of you will find two meals per day more than enough on this plan. If you do drop to two meals you can increase the size of your breakfast by 50 per cent and have it as brunch – or just have lunch and evening meal as suggested.

Eating in the office

Most of the meals in the plan can be made before you go to work and taken to the office in a lunchbox. Even better though is taking them in a large jar which, if stacked properly, helps keep things fresh and crunchy. In this case stack them as follows:

- Place the protein at the bottom of the jar.
- Then add the fat and any dressing.
- Serve the hardiest vegetables next (for example green beans, celery, cabbage, fennel, artichokes, broccoli, cherry tomatoes, beetroot).
- Then add more fragile vegetables like lettuce, rocket, cucumber, kale and chopped tomatoes.
- When you're ready to serve simply tip the contents into a large bowl and mix well.

Takeout lunches that work well

Maybe you don't want to bring lunch to work every day? That's not a problem at all. Here are four suggestions for meals you'll find in most supermarkets or takeaways.

- Any no-carbohydrate salad served with a small portion of extra avocado or nuts

- Portion of vegetable soup with a side portion of salmon, chicken or prawns and a little avocado or a handful of nuts.
- Sashimi, seaweed or edamame salad and a portion of avocado or nuts.
- Two ready-cooked hard boiled eggs, any side salad, portion of nuts.

FIGHTING A SNACK ATTACK

In theory you shouldn't need to snack on this plan. If you do find you're getting hungry or craving sugar though, here are four things to consider:

- Are you still following the rules? If you've started to reduce your fat or protein servings for any reason you could find you're getting hungry. Also, check the labels of any ready-made sauces or foods you're eating. They could contain more sugar than you think and this could be triggering your blood sugar to yo-yo, causing hunger pangs and sugar cravings.

- Are you suffering PMS? Sweet cravings can be common around this time. While it's not definitive, it has been linked to lowered levels of magnesium. Try adding more dark leafy greens to your meals, or try using a magnesium spray before bed (see Appendix 2, page 251). This absorbs into the skin and tops up your supplies – it's also very good for fighting stress and helping sleep.

- Talking of sleep, are you tired? Studies have shown that not getting the hours we need alters levels of our appetite hormones in ways that make us crave more fat and sugar. However, once you get your sleep sorted out that all changes. Trials at the University of Chicago trained poor sleepers to achieve an extra 1.6 hours of sleep a night.

Within two weeks they were eating 14 per cent less food overall – and their cravings for sugary, salty and fatty foods fell by 62 per cent.[30]

- Are you stressed? If you are under any form of stress, be it emotional or physical, this can cause your body to eat into its protein reserves leading to a slight deficiency, which can also cause cravings. If you're stressed, start increasing protein foods in your diet which should counteract this. Also do something relaxing to reduce the stress itself.

MAINTENANCE PLAN RECIPES

BREAKFASTS

Chia porridge (serves one)

25 g (1 oz) chia seeds
60 ml (2.4 fl oz) full-fat milk
25–30 g (1–1.2 oz) blueberries
20 g (0.8 oz) walnuts, crushed
Cinnamon to taste

1 Place the chia seeds in a bowl and add the milk. Stir and leave to sit for five minutes.

2 Stir again being careful to smooth out any lumps. Leave for a further 15 minutes until the seeds swell.

3 Add the blueberries and walnuts. Sprinkle with cinnamon and serve.

Raspberry and walnut parfait (serves one)

60 g (2.4 oz) raspberries
2–3 mint leaves, finely chopped
Juice of half a lime
35 g (1.8 oz) walnuts
150 g (5 oz) Greek yogurt

1 Place the raspberries and mint in a small bowl and gently crush them together, squeeze over a little lime juice.

2 Place the walnuts in a sealed bag and crush them into smaller pieces with a rolling pin.

3 In a tumbler or ice-cream glass, create a bottom layer from one third of the walnuts. Top with one third of the yogurt. Add half the raspberry mixture.

4 Add another layer from one third of the walnuts, and one from another third of the yogurt then add the rest of the raspberries.

5 Add a final layer of yogurt, then top with the last of the walnuts. Add some extra mint as a garnish if you like.

Baked eggs (serves two)

4 eggs
40 ml (1.4 fl oz) double cream
50 g (2 oz) Boursin cheese
3–4 teaspoons pesto
30 g (1.2 oz) pine nuts
4–5 fresh basil leaves

1 Preheat the oven to 160°C/325°F/Gas mark 3.

2 Break the eggs into an oven-proof dish. Pour in the double cream then add the Boursin and pesto, dotting the pesto around the eggs.

3 Bake in the oven for 25 minutes or until the egg whites are cooked through.

4 Garnish with the pine nuts and basil leaves before serving.

LUNCHES AND EVENING MEALS

Steak and feta salad (serves two)

90 g (3.6 oz) lean steak

120 g (4.8 oz) green beans

60 g (2.4 oz) cucumber, chopped

60 g (2.4 oz) red onion

140 g (5.6 oz) avocado, diced

1 teaspoon olive oil

Juice of half a lemon

Handful flat leaf parsley, chopped

90 g (3.6 oz) feta cheese, crumbled

1 Grill or pan-fry the steak for 5–15 minutes depending on your desired level of rareness. Leave to rest for five minutes then slice.

2 Top and tail the green beans then lightly steam for 3–4 minutes. Alternatively, leave them raw for extra crunch.

3 Toss the cucumber, red onion and avocado in a bowl with the olive oil, lemon and parsley. Add the feta and green beans.

4 Divide into two portions to serve and add the sliced steak on top.

Creamy chicken and celery soup (serves two)

2 teaspoons olive oil
180 g (7.2 oz) chicken, diced
450 ml (15 fl oz) chicken stock
120 g (4.8 oz) celery, sliced
1 tablespoon chopped fresh parsley
2 tablespoons single cream

1 Heat the oil in a medium saucepan. Add the chicken and fry for 8–10 minutes until it is cooked through. Remove half the chicken.

2 Add the stock, celery and parsley. Bring to the boil and simmer for 5–10 minutes.

3 While the soup is simmering, chop the reserved cooked chicken into small pieces.

4 Transfer the soup to a food processor and blend until smooth. Pour back into the pan. Add the chicken pieces and warm through. Stir in the cream just before serving. Garnish with any extra parsley.

Peppered lamb steaks with creamy mushroom sauce (serves two)

2 tablespoons mixed peppercorns
1 tablespoon olive oil, plus extra for frying
2 lamb steaks of 140–180 g (5–6.5 oz)
100 g (4 oz) mushrooms, sliced
70 ml (2.8 fl oz) single or double cream

1 Crush the peppercorns using a pestle and mortar and mix with 1 tablespoon of olive oil. Leave to sit.

2 Grill the lamb steaks on one side for 5–8 minutes, depending on your desired level of rareness. Turn, then before placing back under the grill, paint the peppercorn mix on top. Grill for a further 5–8 minutes.

3 Take half the mushrooms and, using a hand blender, blend them together with the cream. Place in a saucepan on a low heat to warm.

4 Pan-fry the leftover mushrooms in a little olive oil.

5 Serve the steaks with sauce on the side and sprinkle the pan-fried mushrooms on top.

Feta and avocado dip (serves two)

2 avocados
80 g (3.2 oz) feta cheese
Juice of half a lemon
½ onion, diced
½ green chilli, chopped and deseeded if preferred
1 handful fresh coriander, chopped

1 Blend the avocado flesh, feta and lemon juice well in a bowl using a hand blender or simply mash them with a fork.

2 Stir in the onion, chilli and coriander.

Creamy ratatouille with grilled salmon
(serves two)

60 g (2.4 oz) aubergine, diced

60 g (2.4 oz) courgette, diced

2 tablespoons olive oil

Salt and pepper, to taste

100 g (4 oz) tinned tomatoes (no added sugar)

1 clove of garlic, crushed

½ teaspoon dried oregano, basil or thyme

Two salmon steaks weighing 150–180 g (5–6.5 oz) each

70 ml (2.8 fl oz) single cream or crème fraîche

1 Fry the vegetables in one tablespoon of olive oil and a pinch of salt until they start to soften.

2 Place in a heavy-bottom saucepan with the tomatoes, remaining olive oil, garlic and herbs.

3 Simmer on a very low heat for 20 minutes.

4 Meanwhile, grill the salmon for 10–15 minutes or until it is cooked through, turning occasionally.

5 Stir the cream into the ratatouille just before serving. Season well then serve the salmon with the ratatouille on top.

Cauliflower bake (serves two)

325 g (11 oz) cauliflower

1 egg, beaten

25 g (1 oz) Parmesan, grated

80 g (3.2 oz) cherry tomatoes, chopped

Salt, pepper and dried oregano, to taste

1 Preheat the oven to 230°C/450°F/Gas Mark 8.

2 Place the cauliflower in a food processor and chop finely. If you're making a smaller amount it can be easier to use the wide holes in a cheese grater.

3 Microwave the cauliflower for 8–10 minutes then place in a sieve with fine holes. Press the cauliflower down with a spoon, you need to remove all the water from it.

4 Mix the cauliflower, egg, cheese and tomatoes in a bowl.

5 Now place in a small, deep ovenproof dish. Bake for 20–25 minutes.

Seafood basmati (serves 2)

100–150 g (4–6 oz) basmati rice

½ teaspoon turmeric

240–280 g (8.5–10 oz) mixed seafood

2 tablespoons of butter or coconut oil

2 cloves garlic, crushed

100–120 g (4–4.8 oz) asparagus

Juice of 1 lemon

Salt and black pepper, to taste

1 Boil the basmati rice as per the instructions, adding the turmeric to the water just before you add the rice.

2 While it cooks, use a wok or large deep-sided frying pan to stir-fry the seafood in the butter and garlic until cooked.

3 Add the asparagus and toss for one minute. Keep everything moving well.

4 Drain the rice and add to the mix, tossing quickly on a high heat just long enough to combine all the ingredients. Add lemon juice, salt and black pepper to taste and serve.

Chicken and black beans (serves two)

150 g (5 oz) dried black beans

1–2 handfuls fresh coriander, chopped

1 clove of garlic, chopped

1 small onion, chopped

1 teaspoon dried cumin

2 teaspoons chilli powder

Salt, to taste

240–480 g (8.5–17 oz) chicken breast

30 g (1.2 oz) sour cream

1 Dried beans need to be soaked before using. The day before you want to make this dish, place the beans in a saucepan and soak them overnight in cold water.

2 Rinse the beans and add to a heavy-bottomed saucepan. Reserve one handful of the coriander but then add the garlic, onion, spices and coriander and salt to the pan. Add enough water to cover the beans and also allow about 1 inch (2.5 cm) liquid on top. Bring to the boil, then turn the heat down as low as you can.

3 Simmer for one to two hours, checking often to check the pan is not boiling dry. If the liquid does start to evaporate, add about a quarter of a cup more water and stir well. Exactly how long the beans will take depends on how well soaked they were, how old they are, the size of the pan and how low you can turn the heat. The beans are done when they are soft to. Drain off any excess liquid if required.

4 When the beans are almost done, grill the chicken. Slice it diagonally. Place the beans on the plate, sprinkle with the reserved coriander then serve with the chicken, and sour cream on the side.

Cod wrapped in Parma ham (serves two)

15 g (0.6 oz) pine nuts

7–10 basil leaves

15 g (0.6 oz) Parmesan cheese

30 ml (1.2 fl oz) olive oil

Half a clove of garlic, crushed

Oil for preparing baking tray

4 slices of Parma ham

2 cod fillets (100–140 g/4–5.6 oz each)

1 Preheat the oven to 180°C/350°F/Gas Mark 4.

2 Put the pine nuts, basil leaves, Parmesan, olive oil and garlic in a bowl and blend with a handheld blender to create a pesto.

3 Oil a baking tray. Divide the Parma ham into two sets of two slices and lay them long sides together, slightly overlapping. Place a cod piece in the middle of each lengthways strip of ham.

4 Add half the pesto mix to each cod steak then wrap the Parma ham over the top to create a parcel.

5 Place the parcels in the oven and cook for 15–20 minutes until the fish is cooked and firm all the way through.

Cauliflower-topped shepherd's pie (serves two)

280–360 g (10–13 oz) beef mince

1 onion, chopped

1 garlic clove, crushed

1 beef Oxo cube, crumbled

100 ml (4 fl oz) beef stock

150 g (5 oz) cauliflower

70 g (2.8 oz) cream cheese

1 Preheat the oven to 200°C/400°F/Gas Mark 6.

2 In a frying pan, fry the beef mince until it starts to brown. Add the onion, garlic and crumble in the Oxo cube. Fry for 2–3 more minutes.

3 Add the beef stock and simmer for 10-12 minutes, then turn the heat up a little until the gravy thickens.

4 Place the beef mixture in the bottom of a small (about 13–18 cm (5–7 inches) in diameter), deep, ovenproof dish.

5 Mash the cauliflower and cream cheese together and smooth on the top.

6 Place in the oven for 20–25 minutes.

DIPS AND SAUCES

Basic peanut butter (makes 10 servings)

450 g (18 oz) peanuts – salted or fresh

1 To make the basic recipe simply put all the peanuts in a food processor and blend. It will take about four minutes to go from chopped nuts to a smooth mixture.

2 It will be warm at this point so spoon it into an airtight jar and allow to cool in the fridge before eating. It will keep for up to two weeks.

VARIATIONS

Chunky peanut butter

Turn the blender off at the chopped nuts-stage and remove 1–2 tablespoons. Then keep blending. Once you've created the butter, add the chopped nuts back in and stir.

Chilli peanut butter

Add half to one teaspoon of chilli powder to the mix as it's blending.

Cinnamon peanut butter

Add half to one teaspoon of cinnamon powder to the mix as it is blending.

STARCHY CARB ALTERNATIVES

The easiest way to replace starchy carbohydrates in your diet is to turn vegetables into carb-like side dishes. They take seconds and work well with all sorts of sauces or as side dishes with any meat, fish or poultry. For each of the methods below on our plan you'll use 50–60 g (2–2.4 oz) per vegetable.

Cauliflower rice

1 Remove all the green parts and wash the florets.

2 Use the large holes on a cheese grater to grate the florets so they look like rice grains. If you are making a large serving you can use a food processor but it doesn't always work so well on smaller portions.

3 Either microwave in a covered dish for 8–10 minutes or sauté using a little olive oil – you can also add chillies, garlic, onion and any herbs or spices to increase the flavour.

4 Need to add some fat to your meal? Adding pine nuts or walnuts gives cauliflower rice a crunchy kick.

Broccoli rice

Use exactly the same method as for the cauliflower rice, but with broccoli you can also use the stalks, they add an extra firmness and are also a good source of added nutrients.

For an extra twist, stir-fry broccoli rice with a little egg to make an egg-fried-rice-style dish.

As with cauliflower rice, adding walnuts or pine nuts gives broccoli rice a crunchy kick.

Courgetti

This works in any dish where you would normally use pasta.

1 Use a spiraliser to turn the courgette into ribbons. If you don't have one you can also use a vegetable peeler to create strips lengthwise.

2 Steam or sauté the ribbons in a little olive oil, butter or coconut oil until they soften. Remember, they are very thin so this won't take long. You don't need a lot of liquid. Use too much and they will go soggy.

3 A simple way to add fat to your meal with courgetti is to toss them in melted cream cheese or crème fraîche just before serving.

C-oodles

If you want a firmer 'noodle' carrots can take more cooking before they start to soften giving slightly more crunch – keeping them as al dente as possible also helps keep their GI low. They work particularly well in stir-fry dishes instead of noodles.

1 Again, you can use a spiraliser or a vegetable peeler for C-oodles.

2 If making a stir-fry, simply add the noodles at the last minute – you want to keep them as close to raw as possible. If you're serving them with a sauce, toss them at the last minute so you are warming them rather than cooking them. Adding a little chilli gives an extra flavour burst.

3 C-oodles work very well with extra cashew nuts, sesame seeds or try melting unsweetened peanut butter with water or coconut milk to make a satay-type sauce.

Alternatives to potatoes

Many vegetables can stand in for potatoes in the form of mash or chips. Mashing vegetables does make them quicker to digest and therefore raises their GI very slightly but it's still far lower than that of mashed potatoes.

Pea mash

This also works well with broccoli and cauliflower.

100–120 g (4–4.8 oz) peas
2–3 fresh mint leaves, chopped
50–70 g (2–2.8 oz) cream cheese

1 Boil the peas as directed – around 4 minutes for fresh, 8–10 for frozen.

2 Place in a bowl with the mint and cream cheese and mash with a fork or potato masher.

Carrot chips (serves two)

2 large carrots, peeled
Olive oil
2 teaspoons Cajun seasoning or dried oregano

1 Preheat the oven to 190°C/375°F/Gas Mark 5.

2 Cut the carrots in half lengthwise, then cut lengthwise again so you end up with four long pieces. Half these in length leaving eight pieces.

3 Brush the carrots with the olive oil and sprinkle with your spice/herb of choice.

4 Place on a lined baking tray and bake for around 30–35 minutes until the carrots are slightly charred round the edges.

Bread alternatives

- Grill thick slices of aubergine and use as an alternative to toast to pile things upon – eat open-sandwich-style with a knife and fork.
- Celery sticks work just like crackers – you can fill them with all manner of fillings from cream cheese and peanut butter to tuna or egg with mayonnaise.
- Lettuce, cabbage or cavolo nero leaves work well as wraps. You can also use sheets of seaweed or strips of mooli for smaller parcels.

DRINK IDEAS

If you're getting a little tired of drinking plain water, then give some of these simple sugar-free blends a try.

Iced coffee

1 Make a cafetière of coffee as normal and leave to cool.
2 Pour the coffee into a tall glass until it is about two-thirds full, then add to a blender with 3–4 ice cubes. Blend until the ice crushes. Add one tablespoon of cream and blend for a further few seconds. Pour the iced mixture back into the glass to serve.

Hot cocoa

1 Brew a cup of the Library Leaves Sweet Treat (which combines cocoa nibs and cinnamon) or Hotel Chocolat Cocoa Infusion (see Appendix 2, pages 250–1). Add hot water and leave to brew for 2–3 minutes.

Iced chocolate

1 Brew a pot of Hotel Chocolat Cocoa Infusion (see Appendix 2, page 250) and leave to cool.

2　Pour into a tall glass until it is two-thirds full, then place in a blender with 3–4 ice cubes. Blend until the ice crushes. Pour the iced mixture back into the glass and top with 1–2 teaspoons of fresh cream.

Fresh mint tea

1　Get 4–5 stalks of fresh mint and crush them between your fingers to release the oil.
2　Place them in a teapot and leave to steep for five minutes.
3　Serve warm, or leave to cool and pour over ice (crushed or cubes).

Cool fruit tea

1　Brew a cup of your favourite fruit or herbal tea.
2　Leave it to cool and pour it over ice.
3　Serve with a sprig of mint.

Chia fresca

1　Pour a large glass of water (you can also use cooled herbal tea).
2　Add one tablespoon chia seeds and leave to rest for five minutes so the chia seeds swell. You can add more chia if you like a thicker drink.
3　Add a dash of lime juice or lemon juice. For true fresca you should now also add a little sugar or sweetener but we're trying to avoid that. If you don't like it without it though, use a little stevia.

Chapter 8

THE 10 RULES FOR STAYING SLIM FOR LIFE

Now you've ended the Maintenance Plan it's time to return to real life. The good news is, it takes 28 days to break an old habit or create a new one and that's how long it's been since you've had sugary foods or snacks, so your reliance on them should now be broken. You've probably also found ways to fill your evening that don't include nibbling in front of the television. And, if you've been doing your visualisation exercises chances are your unconscious now sees your new shape as the picture it thinks is the real you. This all stands you in good stead to keep the weight off for good. But it'll also help to abide by Zana's simple lifelong rules:

1   Get your first meal of the day right. You don't want to start your day spiking insulin. It's very hard to stabilise again if you do and you will be hungry and craving something sweet within a few hours. Breakfast, or the first meal of your day should be a small protein and fat-based one like poached eggs with avocado, bacon and scrambled eggs with butter or natural/Greek yogurt with nuts and some low-GI berries. A study recently published in the *European Journal of Nutrition* found that men eating a breakfast with most of its calories from protein stayed fuller longer and consumed over 300 fewer calories

throughout the rest of the day than those starting their day with a high-carbohydrate meal.[31]

2 Ensure you have some protein with every meal. Depending on your activity level and lifestyle you need approximately 60–120 g (2.2–4.8 oz) in the earlier stage of the day, and 120–180 g (4.8–7.2 oz) in the latter part of the day. On top of this add lots of vegetables (mostly green leafy ones) and about 25–45 g (1–1.8 oz) of fat to all of your meals. If you eat like that 80 per cent of the time, you can relax the rest of the time. Zana's clients generally follow her rules for all their meals during the week and then relax at weekends.

3 Keep very starchy carbs like bread, pasta and rice to just one or two meals a week. Use them as treats not the staple part of every meal. The Maintenance Plan has already shown you how you can enjoy many of your favourites using ideas like vegetable mashes, rices and noodles. Keep using those tricks to keep the GI of your meals as low as you can while still enjoying family favourites.

4 Fats vs carbohydrates. A high-fat plan will not work well with starchy carbohydrates. Combining both fat and carbohydrates consistently and/or excessively is the absolute fastest way to gain weight or increase cholesterol. In other words, don't start eating things like the full-fat cream cheese you've got used to with crackers or toast. On days when you are eating carbohydrates keep the levels of fat in your diet a little lower. If you're not eating carbohydrates it's okay to eat more fat.

5 Alcohol can come back now, but ideally keep it to two days a week. Failing this, at the very least have two days a week when you never touch it. Alcohol itself doesn't cause insulin to rise, but it does seem to bring your body out of any fat-burning state. Alcoholic drinks do contain some carbohydrates – especially beer, sweet wines, cocktails or spirits with any kind of sugary mixer. On top of this, all alcohol contains more calories per gram than

even sugar (seven compared to four) and it can therefore easily create a calorie excess which gets stored as fat. Finally, alcohol also switches off the inhibition parts of the brain making it more likely you'll overindulge. The purer the drink the better, so clear spirits like gin or vodka with soda are considered a better choice than darker or sugary drinks.

6 Don't eat when you're not hungry. We often fall into the habit of eating because it's mealtime – breakfast is a classic example of this. Many people eat it because they have been told it's the most important meal of the day for raising metabolism, but a recent study by experts at the University of Bath found no difference in the number of calories burned per hour in those who ate breakfast compared to those who didn't.[32] The later you eat in the evening, the less likely you are to be hungry the next morning – and vice versa. If you wake up and aren't hungry, don't feel obliged to eat for the sake of it, conversely though if you're hungry, don't skip your morning meal. Listen to your body – it will tell you when it needs to eat.

7 Stop eating when you're full. If we even just followed this rule and the previous one nobody would have a weight problem. Eat without distractions – no television, Internet or social media. Concentrate on how you feel while you're eating and stop when you're full. It's something many of us have forgotten how to do but it should become a habit no matter what is left on your plate. Wait half an hour and if you're still hungry then eat a little more, otherwise don't bother. If you constantly find you're leaving food on your plate then start serving yourself smaller portions.

8 Check for sugar: it's hidden in so many processed foods so if you are going to eat anything you don't make from scratch always, always check the label. Breads, salads, sauces, soups and many other savoury items can all contain sugars. A good rule for day-to-day life is to avoid

all foods with more than 5 g (0.2 oz) of added sugar per 100 g (4 oz) of food. This doesn't mean you can never have dessert, sweets, chocolate or birthday cake, but keep them as treats not a daily eating staple. And, if you return to a point where you start craving sugar or use it to fuel your energy levels, look at your diet or lifestyle (particularly things like stress or lack of sleep as we explain on pages 223–4). Something is affecting your energy negatively, using sugar to prop that up is going to take its toll on your waistline and potentially your health so it's better to find the source than mask the symptom.

9 Keep up the weight training. The more muscle you have, the more you can eat each day and still keep the fat off. Aim to train following the High Intensity Gym Workout – or some other form of high-intensity training – at least three times a week. If you did the High Intensity Home Workout before perhaps think about joining a gym and giving the Gym Workout a try to power up your results. There are schemes now like Pay as You Gym that allow you to join gyms on an ad hoc basis, or, chains like The Gym Group that don't want you to sign up to long-term contracts. At the other end of the scale, for those who live in London, Zana runs three boutique gyms: The Library in Notting Hill and the Little Libraries in Harley Street and Barnes. See thelibrarygym. com for details of membership fees. Also start every day by doing one minute of super-squats (see page 156). They are a very quick way to release a little bit of growth hormone into your system, get your heart and lungs working and fire your metabolism up for the day ahead.

10 Keep an eye on things. Watch inches as opposed to weight, they are a better way of spotting fat creeping back on. If it is, address the issue. It's a lot easier to lose two pounds or a kilo than it is three or four. First go back to ensure you are following rules 1–9 here. If that's not working you may need to try and balance your insulin again so go back

on the 10-Day Blitz. It will work just as well the second time around – remember though, you need to follow it with the same diligence as you did last time.

So that's it – you're all done! Hopefully you're thrilled with your results, and have experienced first hand the value of natural fats, not only in getting you into great shape but also, when combined with as little as 12 minutes of high-intensity exercise, in helping you to stay fit and trim for life.

RECORDING YOUR RESULTS

1) Stand on the scales and record your weight

Starting weight: _____

Finishing weight: _____

2) Measure around your waist at the narrowest point above your tummy button

Starting measurement: _____

Finishing measurement: _____

3) Measure around your tummy at the widest point, usually about 2–5 cm (1–2 in) below your tummy button

Starting measurement: _____

Finishing measurement: _____

4) Measure around the widest part of your hips – this can be lower than you might expect so move the tape measure until you are satisfied it is at the widest point

Starting measurement: _____

Finishing measurement: _____

5) Measure your thigh at the highest point of your leg just underneath your bottom. This is more easily done if you shift most of your weight on to the leg you are measuring causing the muscle of the leg to tense

Starting measurement: _____

Finishing measurement: _____

Starting body fat: _____

Finishing body fat: _____

STOCKISTS

If you're finding it hard to locate some of the things we mention on the plan, or would like Zana's recommendations of the best brands to choose, here are some suggested brands and stockists.

Foods

Chia seeds
Chia Bia at hollandandbarret.com
The Chia Co at nutricentre.com

Cocoa
Hotel Chocolat Cocoa Infusion at hotelchocolat.com

Low-sugar bacon
You can buy completely sugar-free bacon direct from some farms and butchers, otherwise look for brands with less than 0.5g per 100 g like Laverstoke Park Organic Unsmoked Back Bacon at ocado.com

Low-sugar chorizo
Again, go for less than 0.5 g per 100 g which you can find in supermarkets or try boarshead.com
Smaller suppliers do produce both sugar- and nitrate-free chorizo, ask at your local butchers

Japanese peppermint oil
Obbekjaers Oil of Peppermint at nutricentre.com

Protein shakes
Strong Pure Protein Shake at strongnutrients.com

Tea
The Library Leaves Sweet Tea from strongnutrients.com

Supplements

Amino acids
Strong Building Blocks at strongnutrients.com

Creatine
Strong Pure Fine Creatine at strongnutrients.com

Magnesium
Strong Nutrients Magnesium Rocks at strongnutrients.com
Solgar Magnesium Citrate at nutricentre.com

Magnesium spray
BetterYou Magnesium Spray at hollandandbarrett.com
or victoriahealth.com

Multivitamins
Solgar VM2000 at nutricentre.com
Natures Plus Source of Life at nutricentre.com
Quest Once a Day at questexcellence.com

Omega-3
Solgar Omega-3 700 at nutricentre.com
Bare Biology Lion Heart High Strength Capsules at
barebiology.com

Home gym equipment

Resistance bands
Thera-Band Resistance offer multipacks at thera-bands.
co.uk

Yoga mat
yogamatters.com

Other

Ketosis strips
Try Bayer Ketostix at chemistdirect.co.uk or Boots

THE FOOD LISTS AT A GLANCE

During the Pretox

Avoid

- Starchy carbohydrates: bread, pastry, rice, pasta, potatoes, grains, oats, breakfast cereals, etc.
- Sugars: no table sugar, sweets, cakes, chocolate, sweeteners, alcohol
- High-sugar fruits: melon, dates, bananas, figs, grapes, mango, papaya, pineapple, raisins, sultanas

Eat more

- Oily fish, avocados, nuts and occasional high-fat dairy like crème fraîche or cheese

During the 10-Day Blitz

Fats

Allowed

- Dairy foods: butter, clotted cream, crème fraîche, double cream, full-fat cream cheese like Philadelphia or Boursin, mascarpone, single cream, sour cream, whipping cream
- Fruits, nuts and seeds: avocado, CO YO coconut-based yogurt, macadamia nuts, pine nuts, pumpkin seeds, walnuts
- Oils and dressings: all nut oils, coconut oil, homemade mayonnaise, ghee, olive oil – any other liquid oils, except vegetable oil

Avoid

- All nuts not mentioned above: almonds, Brazil nuts, cashews, etc. Any seeds not mentioned above like sunflower or sesame
- Any kind of yogurt
- Fresh coconut, low-fat cream cheese, margarine and low-fat spreads, nut butters, vegetable oils

Proteins

Allowed

- Beef: mince (10 per cent fat or above), ribs (no sauce), steak – particularly rib-eye or sirloin, veal mince
- Cheese: any full-fat cheese like Brie, Camembert, Gorgonzola, Emmental, Gruyère, halloumi, Roquefort, Stilton or blue cheese
- Eggs: organic or free-range. Hen, duck or quail
- Lamb: all cuts including breast, chops, leg, mince, neck, rack, rump, shanks, shoulder
- Oily fish: for example, anchovies, eel, fresh salmon, fresh tuna, herring, kippers, mackerel, pilchards, sardines, smoked salmon, trout, tuna canned in oil, whitebait (not breaded)
- Pork: including bacon particularly streaky bacon (no added sugar and ideally free from nitrates), chorizo (no added sugar and ideally free from nitrates), gammon, pancetta, Parma ham, pork belly, pork chops, pork fillet, ribs (no sauce), tenderloin
- Poultry: chicken drumsticks (skin on), chicken thighs, chicken wings, duck. All chicken should be organic

Allowed with extra fat (cook with butter or oil, eat poultry with the skin on or add cream/cream cheese)

- Beef: less than 5 per cent fat mince, roasting joints, veal
- Dairy: casein protein powder, full-fat cottage cheese,

reduced-fat versions of any cheese including cottage cheese

- Fish: all white fish like cod, haddock, sole, pollock. Tuna canned in brine or spring water
- Offal: liver, kidney, heart
- Pork: lean or reduced-fat mince
- Poultry and game: organic chicken breast, partridge, pigeon, rabbit, turkey, venison
- Shellfish: prawns, mussels, crab, crayfish

Avoid

- Beans and pulses, beefburgers (unless 100 per cent pure beef with no added wheat)
- Breaded fish products
- Canned fish products with any kind of sauce
- Milk and milk products like ice cream
- Processed fish products like crabsticks
- Processed sandwich-style meats, sausages, tinned meats
- Yogurt

Vegetables

Allowed

Alfalfa sprouts, all green lettuce, artichokes, asparagus, aubergine, bamboo shoots, beansprouts, bok choy, broccoli, broccolini, Brussels sprouts, cauliflower, cavolo nero, celery, chilli peppers, courgette, cucumber, edamame, fennel, green beans, green pepper, jalapenos, kale, leeks, marrow, mushrooms, okra, Padron peppers, peas, rocket, runner beans, samphire, savoy cabbage, seaweed, spinach, spring greens, spring onions, Swiss chard, watercress, white cabbage

Avoid

Any vegetables that aren't green or white, and the following that are: root vegetables like celeriac, parsnips, potatoes, radishes, swede. Vegetables that can caramelise like onions or shallots

Herbs, spices, dressings, condiments

Allowed

Any dressings from our recipes. Bay leaves, cayenne pepper, chilli flakes, chilli powder, chives, cinnamon, coriander, cumin, dill, fresh chillies, fresh horseradish, fresh wasabi, garlic, ginger, mint, mustard powder, nutmeg, oregano, paprika, parsley, pepper, rosemary, salt, thyme, turmeric. Lemon juice, lime juice, Tabasco, vinegars like malt, red wine and white

Avoid

Any ready-made rubs or mixes, which may have sugar added. Gravy, fish sauce, ready-made horseradish sauce, ketchup, ready-made mayonnaise, mustard, salad cream, stocks, soy sauce, tartar sauce, vinaigrette

Drinks

Allowed

Black coffee/tea, herbal teas, green tea, hot water and coconut oil, sparkling water, still water, tea/coffee with butter, tea/coffee with coconut oil, tea/coffee with double cream

Avoid

Alcohol, bottled water with sugars, coconut milk, coconut water, fizzy drinks (including diet versions), flavoured milk drinks, juices including vegetable juices, milk, milky coffees, nuts milks, oat milk, probiotic drinks, rice milk, smoothies, soy milk, squashes and cordials, tea with milk

During the Maintenance Plan

Fats

Allowed

- Dairy products: butter, clotted cream, crème fraîche, double cream, full-fat cream cheese, full-fat sour cream, mascarpone, reduced-fat cream cheese, reduced-fat sour cream, single cream, whipping cream
- Fruits: avocado
- Nuts: all types are allowed now. For example, almonds, Brazil nuts, cashews, coconut, hazelnuts, macadamia, peanuts, pecans, pine nuts, pistachios, walnuts
- Nut products: unsweetened CO YO coconut-based yogurt. Unsweetened nut butters
- Seeds: again now you can have any type you like: chia, flax, hemp, linseeds, pumpkin, sesame, sunflower
- Oils: coconut oil, olive oil, any nut oils, ghee, mayonnaise: homemade and ready-made full-fat versions with less than 2 g sugar per 100 g

Avoid

- Margarines and low-fat spreads
- Sweetened nut butters
- Low-fat versions of any foods not specifically listed above
- Vegetable oils

Proteins

Allowed

- Eggs: organic or free-range duck, hen, quail
- Pork: including bacon (no added sugar and nitrate-free), chorizo (no added sugar and nitrate-free), gammon, pancetta, Parma ham, pork belly, pork chops, pork fillet, ribs (no sauce), tenderloin
- Beef: burgers if 100 per cent beef, mince, roasting, ribs

(no sauce), steak – particularly rib-eye or sirloin, veal

- Lamb: all cuts including breast, chops, leg, mince, neck, rack, rump, shanks, shoulder
- Poultry: any organic or free-range chicken – i.e. breast, drumsticks, livers, thighs or wings. Duck, turkey, turkey mince, goose
- Game: venison, rabbit
- Dairy: casein protein powder, full-fat Greek yogurt, reduced-fat Greek yogurt, milk – particularly full fat; any full-fat cheese like Brie, Camembert, Cottage cheese, Gorgonzola, Emmental, Gruyère, halloumi, Roquefort, Stilton or blue cheese
- Fish: all white fish like cod, haddock, sole, pollock, tuna canned in brine or spring water; oily fish such as anchovies, eel, fresh salmon, fresh tuna, herring, kippers, mackerel, pilchards, sardines, smoked salmon, trout, tuna canned in oil, whitebait
- Shellfish: crab, mussels and prawns
- Offal: heart, kidneys, liver
- Vegetable proteins: tofu, TV

Avoid

- Beefburgers that aren't pure beef
- Breaded fish products
- Canned fish products with any kind of sauce
- Non-Greek yogurt of any kind
- Processed fish products like crabsticks
- Processed sandwich-style meats, sausages, tinned meats

Starchy carbohydrates: eat only once or twice a week

Allowed

- Breads: granary bread, rye bread, sourdough, teff bread
- Crackers: oat cakes, rye crackers
- Pasta and noodles: all types of pasta especially if cooked

al dente, glass noodles, kelp noodles, konjac noodles, soba noodles, udon noodles
- Cereals: All Bran, steel-cut oats, unsweetened muesli
- Grains: barley, buckwheat, bulgar wheat, couscous, freekah, quinoa, teff
- Potatoes and tubers: new potatoes, sweet potato, yams
- Rice: basmati rice, brown rice, red rice, wild rice
- Beans and pulses: black beans, butter beans, cannellini beans, chickpeas, kidney beans, lentils, pinto beans, soy beans

Avoid

- Breads: brown breads, white bread of any kind including baguettes, bagels, ciabatta and tortilla wraps
- Crackers: matzo, rice cakes
- Pasta and noodles: gluten-free pasta, rice noodles
- Cereals: any kind of flake, anything with honey, anything with sugar, instant porridge, puffed cereals
- Grains: amaranth, millet
- Potatoes and tubers: any white potato other than new potatoes, mashed sweet potato
- Rice: jasmine rice, quick-cook rice, sticky rice, white rice

Vegetables

Eat daily from this list

Alfalfa sprouts, all lettuce, artichokes, asparagus, aubergine, bamboo shoots, beansprouts, bok choy, broccoli, broccolini, broad beans, Brussels sprouts, cauliflower, cavolo nero, celery, chicory, chilli peppers, courgette, cucumber, edamame, fennel, green beans, green pepper, jalapenos, kale, leeks, marrow, mooli, mushrooms, okra, peas, radish, rocket, runner beans, samphire, savoy cabbage, seaweed, spinach, spring greens, spring onions, Swiss chard, watercress, white cabbage

Enjoy one to two times a week

Beetroot, butternut squash, carrots, celeriac, onions, parsnips, pumpkin, radicchio, red cabbage, red peppers, shallots, turnip, yellow peppers

Fruits

Eat daily

Apples, apricots, blackberries, blackcurrants, blueberries, cherries, grapefruit, harder plums, kiwi, lemon, lime, olives, oranges, peaches, pears, raspberries

Enjoy occasionally

Cantaloupe, grapes, mango, papaya, pineapple, tomato, watermelon. Ripe versions of apricots, peaches, pears, plums, etc.

Avoid

- Any fruit canned in syrup
- Dried fruit like dates, figs, raisins or sultanas
- Juices and smoothies

Herbs, spices, dressings and condiments

Allowed

Bay leaves, capers, cayenne pepper, chilli flakes, chilli powder, coriander, chives, cinnamon, cumin, Dijon mustard, dill, fresh chillies, fresh horseradish, fresh wasabi, garlic, ginger, lemon juice, lime juice, malt vinegar, mint, mustard powder, nutmeg, oregano, Oxo cubes, paprika, parsley, pepper, ready-made pesto, red wine vinegar, rosemary, salt, stock cubes, Tabasco, tapenade, thyme, turmeric, vinegar, white vinegar. Any prepared dressing, rub, sauce or stock with less than 2 g (0.08 oz) sugar per 100 g (4 oz) serving.

Avoid

Agave, balsamic vinegar, BBQ sauce, English mustard, fish sauce, honey, ketchup, mirin, miso, salad cream, soy sauce, sweet chilli sauce, tamari, tomato purée. Any prepared dressing, rub, sauce or stock that has more than 2 g (0.08 oz) of sugar per 100 g (4 oz)

Drinks

Allowed

Black coffee/tea, herbal teas, green tea, hot water with coconut oil, sparkling water, still water, tea/coffee with butter, tea/coffee with coconut oil, tea/coffee with double cream, unsweetened soy or almond milk

Avoid

Alcohol, bottled water with sugars, coconut milk, coconut water, fizzy drinks (including diet versions), flavoured milk drinks, juices including vegetable juices, milky coffees, oat milk, probiotic drinks, rice milk, smoothies, sweetened nut milks, sweetened soy milk, squashes and cordials

THE EXERCISES AT A GLANCE

The Gym Workout

Chest and back

Incline chest press, chest press, seated cable chest press or
standing cable chest press: 3x 6 reps
Pec fly: 3 x 6 reps
Cable pullovers: 3 x 6 reps
Assisted dips: 3 × 6 reps
Lat pulldowns: 3 x 6 reps
Seated row: 3 × 6 reps
Assisted pull-ups: 3x 6 reps
Straight arm pulldown: 3 x 6 reps
Inverted back press: 3 x 6 reps
Press-ups: 30–60 seconds

Shoulders and arms

Shoulder press: 3 x 6 reps
Upright row: 3 x 6 reps
Lateral raise: 3 x 6 reps
Rear deltoid fly (pec deck, cable machine) or rear deltoid
pull: 3 x 6 reps
Bicep curl or cable curl: 3 x 6 reps
Tricep pushdown: 3 x 6 reps
Rope triceps: 3 x 6 reps
Tricep extension: 3 x 6 reps
Bicep curls with free weight: 30 seconds

Tricep dips: 30 seconds
Diamond push-up: 30 seconds

Legs

Leg press or Smith machine squat: 3 x 20 reps
Seated hamstring curl or lying hamstring curl: 3 x 6 reps
Leg extension: 3 x 6 reps
Calf raises (machine or freestanding): 3 x 6, 3 x 12, 3 x 20
Lunges: 60 seconds
Super-squats: 60 seconds

Abdominals

Crunches: 2 x 20
Vertical leg raise: 1 x 20

The Home Workout

Lunges: 60 seconds
Super-squats: 60 seconds
Press-ups: 30 seconds
Seated row: 30 seconds
Lateral raise: 30 seconds
Tricep dips: 30 seconds
Bicep curls: 30 seconds
Diamond push-up: 30 seconds
Calf raises: 3 x 20 seconds
Crunches: 2 x 20
Vertical leg raise: 1 x 20

FURTHER READING

The Big Fat Surprise by Nina Teicholz (Scribe, 2014) explores the science behind why fat may not be as unhealthy as we have been led to think in more detail than we could fit in here. If you want to truly understand the story this is the book to read.

artandscienceoflowcarb.com. Created by research pioneers doctors Jeff Volek and Stephen Phinney. If you want to know anything about the research behind high-fat, low-carbohydrate eating this is where you'll find it.

REFERENCES

1   World Health Organization. Obesity and Overweight Fact sheet No 311 (August 2014)

2   Mintel Dieting UK (February 2004)

3   Grodstein F et al., 'Three-year follow-up of participants in a commercial weight loss program. Can you keep it off?' *Arch Intern Med*, 156 (12) (1996), 1302-1306

4   Greene P, Willet W, Devecis J et al., 'Pilot 12-Week Feeding Weight Loss Comparison. Low-fat vs Low Carbohydrate (Ketogenic) Diets'. Presented at The North American Society for the Study of Obesity Annual Meeting (2003)

5   Norouzy A, Leeds A, Emery P and Bayat I, 'Effect of single high vs low glycemic index (GI) meal on gut hormones'. Presented at the Society for Endocrinology BES Meeting, UK (2009)

6   Shelke K, Mattes R, 'Glycemic index foods at breakfast can control blood sugar throughout the day'. Presented at the Institute of Food Technologists Wellness 12 meeting (2012)

7   Siri-Tarino P, Sun Q, Hu F and Krauss R, 'Meta-analysis of prospective cohort studies evaluating the association of saturated fat with cardiovascular disease'. *Am J Clin Nutr* 91(3) (2010), 535-46

8   Chowdhury R et al., 'Association of dietary, circulating and supplement fatty acids with coronary risk: a systemic review and meta-analysis', *Ann Intern Med.*, (2014), 160(6) 398-406. Erratum in *Ann Intern Med.*, 160 (9) (2014), 658 duly noted

9   Yang Q et al., 'Added Sugar Intake and Cardiovascular Diseases Mortality Among US Adults', *JAMA Intern Med*, 174 (4) (2014), 516-524

10 Yancy W Jr, Olsen M, Guyton J, Bakst R, and Westman E, 'A Low-Carbohydrate, Ketogenic Diet versus a Low-Fat Diet to Treat Obesity and Hyperlipidemia: A Randomized Controlled Trial', *Ann Intern Med.*, 140(10) (2004), 769-777

11 Westman E, Yancy W Jr, Mavropoulos J, Marquart M and McDuffie J, 'The effect of a low-carbohydrate, ketogenic diet versus a low-glycemic index diet on glycemic control in type 2 diabetes mellitus', *Nutr Metab (Lond),* (2008), 5:36

12 Volek J, Sharman M, 'Cardiovascular and hormonal aspects of very-low-carbohydrate ketogenic diets', *Obes Res,* 12 Suppl 2 (2004), 115S-23S

13 Friedman A et al., 'Comparative Effects of Low-Carbohydrate High-Protein Versus Low-Fat Diets on the Kidney', *Clin J Am Soc Nephrol*, 7(7) (2012), 1103-1111

14 Ericson, U et al., 'Food sources of fat may clarify the earlier inconsistent role of dietary fat intake for incidence of type 2 diabetes'. Presented at the European Association for the Study of Diabetes annual meeting (2014)

15 Da Silva M et al., 'Associations between dairy intake and metabolic risk parameters in a healthy French-Canadian population', *Appl Physiol Nutr Metab,* (2014), Sept 16: 1-9

16 Forouhi N et al., 'Differences in the prospective association between individual plasma phospholipid saturated fatty acids and incident type 2 diabetes: the EPIC-InterAct case-cohort study', *Lancet Diabetes Endocrinol.* 2(10) (2014), 810-8

17 Bhutani S, Klempel M, Kroeger C, Trepanowski J, Varady K, 'Alternate day fasting and endurance exercise

combine to reduce body weight and favorably alter plasma lipids in obese humans', *Obesity* (Silver Spring), 21(7) (2013), 1370-9

18   Rudman D et al., 'Impaired growth hormone secretion in the adult population: relation to age and adiposity', *J Clin Invest*, 67(5) (1981), 1361-1369

19   National Diet and Nutrition Survey (2014)

20   Office of National Statistics General Lifestyle Survey

21   National Diet and Nutrition Survey (2014)

22   Annual Report of the Chief Medical Officer, Surveillance Volume (2012)

23   Weigle D et al., 'A high-protein diet induces sustained reductions in appetite, ad libitum caloric intake, and body weight despite compensatory changes in diurnal plasma leptin and ghrelin concentrations', *Am J Clin Nutr.* 82(1) (2005), 41-8

24   Suez J et al., 'Artificial sweeteners induce glucose intolerance by altering the gut microbiota', *Nature*, 514(7521) (2014), 181-6

25   Simic L, Sarabon N, Markovic G, 'Does pre-exercise static stretching inhibit maximal muscular performance? A meta-analytical review', *Scand J Med Sci Sports*, 23 (2) (2013), 131-48

26   Gergley J, 'Acute effect of passive static stretching on lower-body strength in moderately trained men', *J Strength Cond Res*, 27(4) (2013), 973-7

27   Bauer P, Pivarnik J, Feltz D, Paneth N and Womack C, 'Relationship of Past-Pregnancy Physical Activity and Self-efficacy With Current Physical Activity and Postpartum Weight Retention', *Am J Lifesty Med*, 8 (1) (2014), 68-73

28   Ranganathan V, Siemionow V, Liu J, Sahgal V and Yue G, 'From mental power to muscle power – gaining strength by using the mind', *Neuropsychologia*, 42(7) (2004), 944-56

29   Wood J, Perunovic W, Lee J, 'Positive self-statements:

power for some, peril for others', *Psychol Sci.*, 20(7) (2009), 860-6

30 Tasali E, Chapotot F, Wroblewski K and Schoeller D, 'The effects of extended bedtimes on sleep duration and food desire in overweight young adults: A home-based intervention', *Appetite*, 80 (2014), 220-4

31 Fallaize R, Wilson L, Gray J, Morgan L and Griffin B, 'Variation in the effects of three different breakfast meals on subjective satiety and subsequent intake of energy at lunch and evening meal', *Eur J Nutr*, 52(4) (2013), 1353-9

32 Betts J, Richardson J, Chowdhury E, Holman G, Tsintzas K and Thompson D, 'The causal role of breakfast in energy balance and health: a randomized controlled trial in lean adults', *Am J Clin Nutr*, 4:100(2) (2014), 539-547

ACKNOWLEDGEMENTS

Zana: My sincerest thanks to Helen and Nancy Brady, for gently strong-arming me and without whom there would be no book. To the incredibly talented Nicola Bensley for the most stunning pictures, not to mention her patience and flexibility. To the amazing Alex Howard, for making so many of my clients so, so happy with her beautiful recipes. The entire team of The Library Gym, whose diligence over the years has allowed us to develop and evolve. To Tony Quinn for his inspiration and teachings, and my family for theirs. Maggie Lawrie and Catherine Cherrington for their endless patience and support. And finally, to Karen Welman, the Alchemist, for her endless impatience, constant fun and never letting me off the hook. Thank you.

Helen: Thanks firstly to Zana for finally ending my battles with my body – and giving in to my nagging to let the rest of the UK hopefully do the same – and to Nancy Brady for helping persuade her. Thanks to Brigid Moss without whom we would never have met the fabulous team at Random House. And to all the lovely editors who let me have the time off to write this without nagging me – particularly Kate Minogue, Lucy Elkins, Anna Magee, Lara Nugent and Sarah Gooding who all moved things around to make it happen. I'd also like to thank the esteemed scientists who kindly gave me permission to specifically mention their work in this complicated field in this book: Dr Uffe Ravnskov, Dr Stephen Phinney, Dr William Yancy, Dr Eric Westman and

Dr Jeff Volek. Finally, a special mention has to go to Neil who dealt with all the hysterical meltdowns as deadlines got nearer – and to Luella Forbes and Arian Vitali for their friendship even though they are a million miles away. You're in a book, ladies.

INDEX

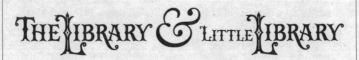
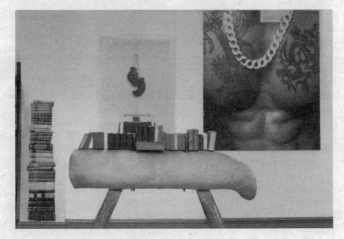